SURVIVAL

HERBS, FOODS, TREATMENTS AND PREPARATIONS

M. Susan Thuillard

authorHOUSE

AuthorHouse™
1663 Liberty Drive
Bloomington, IN 47403
www.authorhouse.com
Phone: 833-262-8899

Published by AuthorHouse 07/30/2021

ISBN: 978-1-6655-3314-0 (sc)
ISBN: 978-1-6655-3313-3 (e)

This is a compilation of tried and tested methods in using natural ingredients and remedies for life's 'bumps and bruises' or illnesses, or even nutritional food products and much more. These recipes and methods have been developed and/or organized by the author over years of use. Any similarities to other recipes and methods is purely coincidental.

- M. Susan Thuillard

INTRODUCTION

I have lived in several places and talked to many people throughout my life. Everyone, it seems has a tradition of herbal lore that has been passed down through their families or their peoples. I have tried many of them and found some success in varied uses for the earth's abundance.

Reading in the Bible and other religious books, I have discovered that the Lord provided for the people of the earth a cornucopia of plants and herbs that would be useful. Some can be eaten, others taken for ailments, and some are good for both.

There is seemingly no end to the uses we can find for the plants of the earth. They are as varied as the plants themselves. There are however, some guidelines and common sense rules to using wild plants and common weeds so as not to do the wrong thing. Some plants can be toxic when used improperly and others are deadly and shouldn't be used at all without sure and certain knowledge.

I have put together this guide for the use of plants from varying climes and areas. It must be noted that medicinal use of plants does not guarantee success. We are all made up differently and may have odd reactions to herbs and plants that work quite well for others. Or, we may have no reaction at all. It is also recommended that a person not use natural medicinal herbs in place of prescriptions for many diseases and disorders at advanced stages. Using medicinal herbs with prescription drugs can bring on reactions that could be harmful. Make sure to tell your doctor and get advice about the use of medicinal herbs and plants.

Also are included foods and methods to produce foods from your own resources in the form of domesticated and wild meats including canning, tanning, and processing for survival and/or independent living ("off the grid").

Above all else, have fun finding the things that work for you, and that taste good or improve your healthy lifestyle.

The Author, M. Susan Thuillard

PART ONE
MEDICINES AND AILMENTS

QUICK GUIDE TO A FEW USEFUL PLANTS

HERB OR PLANT	USE
Aloe Vera	Sap for burns, rashes, and bug bites
Apple Bark	Tea for Fever
Aspen Bark	Tea for headaches, itches, pains, etc.
Birch Bark	Tea for antiseptic or internally for diarrhea
Black Cohosh Bark	Tea for cramps and as a sedative
Burdock	Salve for burns and boils
Cattails	Bandaging, antiseptic / edible tubers
Chia Seeds	Add to foods to boost energy, stamina
Cobwebs	To staunch bleeding.
Comfrey	Poultice for antiseptic, tea for cough/chest problems
Dandelion Root	Decoction for a diuretic
Mullein	Tea for allergies, to calm nerves, and to sleep
Marshmallow	Tea for douching and to replace bodily fluids
Nettle	Tea to expel worms
Peppermint	Tea for colds, flu, aches, nausea and vomiting
Plantain Leaves	Poultice for sprains, bruises, and swelling
Puffball	Powder to staunch bleeding and promote healing
Raspberry Leaf	Tea for infant diarrhea
Red Clover Blossom	Tea to calm nerves
Sassafras Root	Poultice for chest complications (pleurisy)
Strawberry Leaf	Stings, bug bites, etc.
Strawberry Root	Nausea and cramps

"MEDICINES"

AILMENT	HERB	PORTION	PREPARATION
A			
Aches	Peppermint	Leaves	Tea
	Juniper	Berries	Crush and Apply Directly
	Poplar	Inner Bark	Tea
Appendicitis	Vervain	Whole Plant	Tea
	Lady's Slipper	Whole Plant	Tea (Cleanse, Laxative)
Acne	Calendula (Marigold)	Petals	Infusion (Cleanser)
Anemia	Comfrey	Root	Tea
	Dandelion	Leaves	Greens (Eat)
	Raspberry	Leaves	Tea
Allergies	Chamomile	Roots, Flowers	Crush to Powder (Capsule)
	Mullein*	Leaves	**Mild T**ea
Alzheimer's	Gingko	Commercial	Capsules
	Rosemary	Leaves	Tea
Anxiety	Willow	Inner Bark, Root	Tea
Athlete's Foot	Tea Tree Oil	Commercial	Apply
Antiseptic	St. John's Wort	Flowers	Salve
	Garlic	Pod	Poultice
	Comfrey	Leaves	Bruised, Apply Directly
	Plantain	Leaves	Bruised, Apply Directly
	Thyme	Leaves	Infusion
	Birch	Leaves, Inner Bark	Oil, Apply Directly
	Burdock	Flowers, Leaves	Salve
	Tree Fungus	Pulp	Apply Directly
	Pine	Sap, Naturally Dried	Apply Directly as a Bandage
Astringents	Bearberry	Leaves	Infusion
Arthritis	Ginger	Root	Tea
	Turmeric	Root	Tea
	Willow	Inner Bark, Root	Tea
	Pineapple Enzyme	Commercial	Pill Form
	Papaya Enzyme	Commercial	Pill Form
	Yucca	Root	Tea
	Devil's Claw	Root	Tea
	Indian Frankincense	Commercial	Pill Form

AILMENT	HERB	PORTION	PREPARATION
B			
Bad Breath	Anise	Seeds	Tea (Rinse)
Bronchitis	Echinacea	Commercial	Capsule
Burns	St. John's Wort	Flowers	Salve
	Burdock	Roots, Leaves	Salve
	Chickweed	Leaves	Salve
	Comfrey	Root	Poultice
	Allow Vera	Sap	Apply Directly
	Plantain	Leaves	Tea (Swab)
Boils	Burdock	Leaves	Tea (Swab)
	Tea Tree Oil	Commercial	Apply Directly
	Comfrey	Root	Fomentation
	Red / White	Blossoms	**Strong** Tea (Apply Directly)
	Clover	Plant **and**	Poultice,
	Lobelia* **and**	Inner Bark	(Ratio - 1/3:2/3)
	Slippery Elm	Leaves, Inner Bark	Oil (Apply Directly)
	Birch		
Bed Wetting	Sweet Corn	Silk	Eat Raw
Brain Function	Chia	Seeds	Eat Raw or Cooked in Foods

AILMENT	HERB	PORTION	PREPARATION
C			
Cough	Anise	Seeds	Syrup
	Marshmallow	Plant	Syrup
	Comfrey	Root	Tea
	Rosemary	Leaves, Flowers	Tea
	Ginseng	Root	Tea
	Flax	Linseed Oil	Flavoring
	Hyssop	Leaves	Infusion
Colds	Garlic	Cloves	Syrup or Eat Raw
	Ginger	Root	Tea
	Echinacea	Commercial	Capsules
	Peppermint	Leaves	Tera
	Sage	Leaves	Tea
	Nettle	Green Leaves	Tea
	Summer Savory	Whole Plant	Tea
	Vervain	Whole Plant	Tea
	Yarrow	Root	Tea, Syrup
Chest Trouble	Ginseng	Root	Flavored Drink
	Yarrow	Plant	Tea
	Sassafras	Root, Bark	**Warm** Tea
	Mullein*	Leaves	**Mild** Tea
		Flowers	
Convulsions	Pennyroyal**	Whole Plant	Tea
	Peppermint	Leaves	Tea
Cramps	Cayenne	Powder	Capsule
	(Stomach)	Whole Plant	Fomentation
	Thyme	Root	Fomentation
	Black Cohosh	Flowers	**Medium Steeped** Tea
	Hibiscus		
Cancer	Clover	Blossoms	Strong Tea
Sores-	Sage	Root	**Mild** Tea (Wash)
Prostate-	Cucumber	Seeds	Eat
	Pumpkin	seeds	Eat
Cankers	Goldenseal	Root	Tea (Wash)
	Peroxide	Commercial Liquid	Capful (Swish in Mouth)
Cerebral Circulation	Ginko Biloba	Commercial	Capsule
Cuts	Comfrey	Leaves	Bruised, Apply Directly
	St. John's Wort	Flowers	Ointment
	Pine	Sap, naturally dried	Apply Directly as Bandage

Cirrhosis	Milkweed	Root	Tea
Colitis	Peppermint	Leaves	Tea
Cystitis	Cranberry	Berries	Dried and Crushed to Powder (Capsule)
Constipation	Chickweed Ginger Rhubarb Peach	Leaves Powder Root Leaves	Tea Tea Tea Tea
Chapped lips, rash	Chickweed	Leaves	Salve, Apply Directly

AILMENT	HERB	PORTION	PREPARATION
D			
Depression	Lavender	Flowers	Tea
	Hibiscus	Flowers	**Mild** Tea
Disinfectant	Goldenseal	Leaf	Bruised, Apply
		Root	Powdered, Apply
Diuretic	Dandelion	Root	Decoction
	Marshmallow	Whole Plant	Decoction
Diabetes II	Garlic	Cloves	Eat
	Hibiscus	Berries	Eat, Tea
Diabetes	Goldenseal	Root	Tea
	Dandelion	Root	Tea
	Marshmallow	Root	Tea
	Blueberry	Berry, Leaves	Eat, Tea
	Raspberry	Leaves	Tea
	Cinnamon	Powder, Stick	Add to Foods, Swirl in Tea or Other Drinks
Dyspepsia	Ginger	Root	Tea
	Chamomile	Root	Tea
Dandruff	Sage	Leaves	Tea as Hair Tonic
Diverticulitis	Peppermint	Leaves	Tea
Diarrhea	Birch	Inner Bark	Tea
	Comfrey	Roots	Tea
	Peppermint	Leaves	Tea
	Strawberry	Leaves	Tea, Eat Raw
	Raspberry	Leaves	Tea, Eat Raw
	Edelweiss	Whole Plant	Tea
Dementia	Rosemary	Leaves	Tea, Add to Foods
	Medical Marijuana	Oil	In foods or as "gummies"

AILMENT	HERB	PORTION	PREPARATION
E			
Eczema	Chamomile	Root	Tea (Drink / Bathe)
Encephalitis	Garlic	Root	Tea
Earache	Lemon	Juice	Drops (Warm)
	Mullein*	Flower Head	Oil Drops (Warm)
	Garlic	Cloves	Oil Drops (Warm)
Endurance, Energy	Chia	Seeds	Eat, Cook Into Foods

AILMENT	HERB	PORTION	PREPARATION
F			
Fever	Sage	Leaves	Strong Tea
	Vervain	Whole Plant	Tea
	Apple Tree	Inner Bark	Tonic
	Parsley	Leaves	Weak Tea
	Lobelia*	Plant	Tea (Infusion)
	Borage	Young Leaves	Infusion
	Pennyroyal**	Whole Plant	Tea (Poultice)
	Poplar	Inner Bark	Tea
Flu	Echinacea	Commercial Powder	Capsules
	Peppermint	Leaves	Tea
	Poplar	Leaves, Inner Bark	Tea
	White Pine	Inner Bark	Tea
	Burdock	Leaves	tea

AILMENT	HERB	PORTION	PREPARATION
G			
Gas	Peppermint	Leaves	Tea
	Sage	Leaves	**Strong** Tea
	Strawberry	Leaves	Eat, Tea
	Fennel	Seeds	Tea
	Gripe Water	Commercial	Syrup for Babies (Colic)
Gallstones	Milkweed	Root	Tea
	Parsley	Leaves, root	**Weak** Tea
	Rhubarb	Root	Tea
Gingivitis	Goldenseal	Root	Tea (Wash)
Gangrene	Comfrey	Root	Poultice
	Poplar	Inner Bark	Wash
	Charcoal	Powder	Poultice
Gargle	Goldenseal	Root	Powder (Dissolve in Water)
	Sage	Leaves	**Strong** Tea
	Fennel	Seeds	Tea
	Garlic	Cloves	Tea
Gout	Nettle	Root	Tea
	Celery	Seeds	Eat as seasoning
	Alfalfa	Leaves	Add to salad or other foods
	Birch	Inner bark	Tea
	Willow	Inner bark	Tea

AILMENT	HERB	PORTION	PREPARATION
H			
High Blood Pressure	Borage	Leaves	Tea
Hay Fever	Nettles	Root	Tea
Hepatitis	Milkweed	Root	Tea
HIV	Echinacea	Commercial	Capsule
Hot Flashes	Red Clover	Blossoms	Tea
	Soy	Oil	Swallow
	Garlic	Cloves	Eat
Heart Problems	Goldenseal	Root	Tea
	Peppermint	Leaves	Tea
Headache	Peppermint	Leaves	Tea
	Rhubarb	Root	Tea
	Thyme	Whole Plant	Tea
	Lavender	Flower, Stem	Cold Compress
	Pennyroyal	Whole Plant	Tea
	Rosemary	Leaves, Flower	Tea
	Ginger	Root	Tea (Compress)
	Poplar	Inner Bark	Tea
Hemorrhoids	Burdock	Leaves	Salve, Apply Directly
	Goldenseal	Root	Tea (Drink, Wash)
	Edelweiss	Root	Capsule
Hemorrhage	Comfrey	Root	Tea
	Nettle	Whole Plant	Decoction
	Yarrow	Whole Plant	Enema
	Plantain	Leaves	Tea (Suppository)

AILMENT	HERB	PORTION	PREPARATION
I			
Itching	Lemon	Juice	Apply Directly
Indigestion	Watercress	Leaves, Stems	Infusion
	Spearmint	Leaves	Hot Infusion
	Alfalfa	Flowers, Leaves	Tea
	Bay	Leaves	Tea
Inflammation	Sage	Leaves	Poultice
	Calendula (Marigold)	Petals	Infusion
Infection	Goldenseal	Root	Powder, Capsule
	Tea Tree Oil	Commercial	Swallow, Apply Directly
Influenza	Peppermint	Leaves	Tea
	Poplar	Leaves, Inner Bark	Tea
	White Pine	Inner Bark	Tea
	Burdock	Leaves	Tea
	Echinacea	Commercial	Capsule
Insect Bites	Parsley	Leaves	Fomentation
	Plantain	Green Leaves	Bruise, Apply Directly
	Pennyroyal**	Whole Plant	Poultice / Tea (Wash to Repel Insects)
Insomnia	Mullein*	Flowers	Tea
	Peppermint	Leaves	**Strong** Tea
	Valerian*	Root	Tea
Ivy Poison	Goldenseal	Root	Crush (Apply Directly, Damp)
	Beech Tree	Inner Root	Tea (Wash)

AILMENT	HERB	PORTION	PREPARATION
J			
Jock Itch	Lemon	Juice	Wash

AILMENT	HERB	PORTION	PREPARATION
K			
Kidney Problems	Quack Grass	Roots	Tea
	Bearberry	Leaves	Tea
	Borage	Young Leaves	Infusion
	Hibiscus	Flowers	**Mild** Tea
Kidney Stones	Juniper	Berries	Tea, Eat Raw
	Goldenrod	Flowers	Tea

AILMENT	HERB	PORTION	PREPARATION
L			
Lactation	Basil	Leaves	Tea
	Marshmallow	Leaves	Tea
Lactation, dry up	Cabbage	Leaves	Apply directly to breasts and bind
Laxative	Goldenseal	Roots	Tea
	Mullein*	Leaves	Crush, Milk Tea
	Sage	Leaves	**Strong** Tea
	Borage	Young Leaves	Infusion
	Hibiscus	Flowers	**Strong** Tea
Liver Function	Hibiscus	Flowers	**Mild** Tea

AILMENT M	HERB	PORTION	PREPARATION
Measles	Yarrow Raspberry Burdock	Whole Plant Leaves Leaves	Tea Tea (Drink, Wash) Infusion
Migraines	Valerian* Medical Marijuana	Root Oil	**Mild** Tea Eat as "gummies" or in foods
Mouthwash	Goldenseal	Leaves	Tea (Swish Orally)
Motion Sickness	Ginger	Root	Tea (Before Riding)
Myalgia (muscle pain)	Wintergreen	Oil	Ointment
Multiple Sclerosis	Chamomile Valerian Medical Marijuana	Leaves Root Leaves, Oil	Tea Tea Vape, Eat in 'gummies' or foods

AILMENT N	HERB	PORTION	PREPARATION
Nausea	Ginger Peppermint Red Raspberry Pennyroyal** Lobelia*	Roots Leaves Leaves Whole Plant Leaves	Tea Tea Tea Tea Tea
Nose, Plugged	Eucalyptus	Leaves	Oil, Apply Directly or Inhale in Steam
Nervousness	Celery Dill Red Clover Lobelia* Chamomile Valerian*	Root, seeds Seeds Flower Whole Plant Leaves Root	Eat Eat Tea **Mild** Tea Tea **Mild** Tea

AILMENT	HERB	PORTION	PREPARATION
O			
Osteoporosis	Nettle	Root	Tea
Oak Poison	Beech	Inner Bark	Tea, Wash
Obesity	Hibiscus	Flowers	**Medium Steeped** Tea

AILMENT	HERB	PORTION	PREPARATION
P			
Pneumonia	Marshmallow	Leaves, Roots	**Cool** Tea
	Sage	Leaves	**Strong** Tea
	Comfrey	Root	Tea
	Willow	Inner Bark	tea
Pimples	Plantain	Whole Plant	Bruise, Apply Directly
			Tea (Wash)
	Calendula	Petals	Salve, Apply Directly
	(Marigold)	Leaves	Infusion, Ointment
	Hibiscus		Bruise, Apply Directly
Pain	Mullein*	Flowers	Tea
	Nettle	Green Leaves	Poultice
	Dill	Seeds	Eat Raw
Pain, Muscular	Hyssop	Leaves	Compress
	Lavender	Flowers, Stems	Infusion
pleurisy	Marshmallow	Leaves, Roots	**Cool** Tea
	Sage	Leaves	**Strong** Tea
	Comfrey	Root	Tea
	Willow	Inner Bark	Tea
Parkinson Disease	Chamomile	Leaves	Tea
	Valerian	Root	Tea
	Medical Marijuana	Leaves, Oil	Vape, Eat in 'gummies' or foods

AILMENT	HERB	PORTION	PREPARATION
Q			
Quaking	Celery	Root, Seeds	Eat
	Red Clover	Flower	Tea
	Chamomile	Leaves	Tea
	Medical Marijuana	Leaves, Oil	Vape, Eat in "gummies" or foods

AILMENT	HERB	PORTION	PREPARATION
R			
Ringworm	Yellow Dock	Leaves	Tea (Wash)
	Burdock	Leaves	Infusion
Rheumatism	Cabbage	Leaves	Ironed Leaf Poultice
Rush	Calendula (Marigold)	Whole Plant	Ointment
	St. John's Wort	flowers	Salve
Rupture	Comfrey	Root	Poultice

AILMENT S	HERB	PORTION	PREPARATION
Skin Disease Includes Ringworm	Burdock Dandelion Sassafras Plantain Pennyroyal**	Leaves, Root Root Root, Bark Leaves Whole Plant	Salve or Infusion Tea Tea (Wash) Pound to a Paste, Apply Directly Poultice
Sores, Open	Plantain Carrots Burdock	Leaves Root Leaves	Poultice, Bruise and Apply Fresh Directly Grated Raw, Poultice Poultice
Sores, Mouth	Pennyroyal** Garlic	Whole Plant Pod	Tea (Swish) Poultice
Swelling	Plantain	Leaves	Bruised, Apply Directly
Scars	Calendula (Marigold)	Petals	Ointment
Snake Bite	Pennyroyal** Plantain	Whole Plant Whole Plant	Tea (Swish), Poultice Poultice
Sinuses	Eucalyptus	Leaves	Tea (Wash) Poultice
Sprains	Comfrey Calendula (Marigold)	Root Petals	Fomentation Bruise, Apply Directly
Sore Throat	Cayenne Ginger Mullein* Peroxide	Powder Root Flowers Liquid	Capsule Chew Tea Gargle
Sleep Inducer	Mullein* Peppermint Valerian*	Flowers Leaves Root	Tea **Strong** Tea Tea
Seizures	Chamomile Valerian Medical marijuana	Leaves Root Leaves, Oil	Tea Tea Vape, Eat in 'gummies' or foods

AILMENT	HERB	PORTION	PREPARATION
T			
Tumors	Nettle	Leaves	Poultice
	Mullein*	Leaves	Poultice
Toothache	Sassafras	Leaves	Oil, Apply Directly
	Cloves	Pod	Oil, Apply Directly
	Summer Savory	Leaves	Oil, Apply Directly
	Yarrow	Whole Plant	Infusion
	Willow	Root	Powdered, Apply as a Paste
	Pennyroyal**	Whole Plant	Tea
	Plantain	Root	Powdered, Apply as a Paste
Tonsilitis	Goldenseal	Leaves	Tea (Gargle)
Tooth Cutting Pain	Marshmallow	Root	Tea (Rub on Gums)
Tremors	Medical Marijuana	Leaves, Oil	Vape or Eat in foods or as "gummies"

AILMENT	HERB	PORTION	PREPARATION
U			
Ulcers	Alfalfa	Flowers, Leaves	Tea
	Licorice	Commercial	Eat

AILMENT	HERB	PORTION	PREPARATION
V			
Vaginal Douche	Marshmallow	Leaves	**Warm** Tea, Wash
	Kinnickinnick	Leaves	**Warm** Tea, Wash
	Raspberry	Leaves	**Warm** Tea, Wash
	Goldenseal	Root	**Warm** Tea, Wash
Vaginitis	Goldenseal	Leaves	**Warm** Tea, Wash
Vertigo	Ginko Biloba	Commercial	Capsules
	Ginger	Root	Tea or Capsules
Vomiting	Clover	Blossoms	Tea
Vericose Veins	Edelweiss	Root	Capsules

AILMENT	HERB	PORTION	PREPARATION
W			
Warts	Mullein*	Fresh Flowers	Crush, Apply Directly
	Milkweed	Pod Milk	Apply Directly
Worms	Birch	Inner Bark	Tea
	Nettle	Whole Plant	Tea
	Sage	Leaves	**Strong** Tea
	Poplar	Leaves, Inner Bark	Tea
	Carrot	Root	Juice, Drink
	Cabbage	Leaves	Juice, Drink
	Fennel	Seeds	Tea
Wounds	Plantain	Leaves	Bruise, Apply Directly
	Goldenrod	Leaves	Powdered, Apply Directly as
	Solomon Seal	Root	Paste
	Cattail	Heads	Poultice
	Tree Fungus	Pulp	Bandaging
	Garlic	Cloves	Apply Directly
			Compress
Weakness	Borage	Leaves	Tea
	Poplar	Inner Bark	Decoction
Weight Loss / Control	Hibiscus	Flowers	**Medium Steeped** Tea

AILMENT	HERB	PORTION	PREPARATION
X			

AILMENT	HERB	PORTION	PREPARATION
Y			
Yeast Infection	Garlic	Root	Eat
	Goldenseal	Root	**Warm** Tea, Wash
	Marshmallow	Leaves	**Warm** Tea, Wash

AILMENT	HERB	PORTION	PREPARATION
Z			

*Be careful of the strength of the tea as it may cause deep, prolonged sleep.

**DO NOT give to pregnant women (may cause miscarriage).

Psychological or Emotional Disorders

DISORDER	HERB	PORTION	PREPARATION
Anxiety	Willow	Inner Bark, Root	Tea
	Hawthorn	Berry	Salve for bottoms of feet
	Medical Marijuana	Leaves, Oil	Vape, eat in foods or as "gummies"
BI-polar -Manic Bi-polar -Depressive	Willow	Inner Bark, Root	Tea
	Hawthorn	Berry	Salve for bottoms of feet
	Lavender	Flowers	Tea
	Hibiscus	Flowers	**Mild** Tea
		Berry	Salve for bottoms of feet
Depression	Lavender	Flowers	Tea
	Hibiscus	Flowers	**Mild** Tea
		Berry	Salve for bottoms of feet
Hyperactivity	Hawthorn	Berry	Salve for bottoms of feet
	Celery	Stalks, Seeds	Eat
	Red Clover	Flower	Tea
	Chamomile	Leaves	Tea
Nervousness	Celery	Stalks, Seeds	Eat
	Dill	Seeds	Eat
	Red Clover	Flower	Tea
	Lobelia*	Whole Plant	**Mild** Tea
	Chamomile	Leaves	Tea
	Valerian*	Root	**Mild** Tea
Paranoia	Lobelia*	Whole Plant	**Mild** Tea
	Valerian*	Root	**Mild** Tea
	Celery	Stalks, Seeds	Eat
Sleep Disorder	Mullein*	Flowers	Tea
	Peppermint	Leaves	**Strong** Tea
	Valerian*	Root	Tea

*Be careful of the strength of the tea as it may cause deep, prolonged sleep.

**DO NOT give to pregnant women (may cause miscarriage).

ALTERNATIVE THERAPIES

Tuning forks and the Tibetan Singing Bowl have been used for calming and restorative therapies for centuries. You can obtain your own instruments from several vendors over the internet, at low cost. Tuning forks have traditionally been used to test hearing and to ascertain if bones have been cracked or broken when more sophisticated instruments are not available. Tuning forks waved over the head and body for the vibrations can improve mental clarity and renew physical energy. The Tibetan Bowl requires some skill that can be developed with practice. The sweet tones are used to calm the mind during meditation or quiet reflection. The tones may also support deep muscle relaxation and regeneration, relieve joint and spinal pain, improve cognition and digestion.

Our senses are attuned to the earth. We feel different depending on the Phases of the Moon and the Barometric Pressure. Touch, Smell, Taste, Hearing, and Sight are individually and uniquely important in our life. Even if we have a lack of one or more of the basic senses, we develop a keener awareness in other senses and cope with life in our own, unique ways. Certain stones can influence healing properties within our bodies. There are areas of the body (Chakra) that are sensitive to these stones, light, tone, and aroma when all used together.

Color has more influence than just sight. Different colors may affect our moods in a multitude of ways. Some are soothing and others exciting. Knowing the right blend of colors for your own aura is important to your peace and serenity.

Smell is affected and assaulted in many ways every day. We can use aromas to alter or heal our moods and other senses.

Putting it altogether:

Symptom/ Condition	Chakra/ Color/Aura	Body Area/ Stone	Tone	Aroma	Feeling
Anxiety, Digestion, Breathing, Immune	#1 / Red / Survival	Base of Spine "Root" Ruby or Obsidian	G	Frankincense, Myrrh	Security, Warmth
Anxiety, Breathing, Dementia	#2 / Orange / Pleasure	Lower Abdomen Naval Amber	A	Tea Tree	Cleansing, Warmth
Headache, Cold/ Flu, Circulation, Focus	#3 / Yellow / Power	Solar Plexus Citrine Topaz	A#	Eucalyptus, Rosemary	Willpower, Balance
Arthritis, Insomnia, Muscle soreness, Circulation	#4 / Green / Love	Heart Rose Quartz	Middle C,	Citron, Hyssop, Lavender, Peppermint	Refreshed, Clean, Warmth
Arthritis, Dementia, Headache, Anxiety	#5 / Blue / Awakening	Throat Aquamarine	D	Citronella, Peppermint, Pine	Refreshed, Positive Energy
Depression, Mental Fatigue	#6 / Indigo / Wisdom	Third Eye/ Middle of Forehead Indigo Tourmaline	D#	Chamomile, Peppermint	Relaxed, Imagining
Insomnia, Headache, Depression	#7 / Violet or White / Divine or Complete	Crown of Head Clear Quartz	E	Lavender, Pine, Chamomile	Refreshed, Spiritual Maturity

Colored Light and Tone Therapies for Specific Conditions:

Condition	Tone	Color Technique
Alcohol Addiction	D,G,G#+D	Blue and Magenta on Systemic Front, Scarlet on Systemic Front and Systemic Back if blood circulation is weak.
Alzheimer's Disease	B,G+E	Lemon on Systemic Front, Magenta on Crown, Throat, Chest, and Navel.
Blood Pressure-High	B,A#+E	Lemon and Purple on Systemic Front and Systemic Back or Whole Body Front and Whole Body Back, Magenta on Chest and Navel.
Blood Pressure-Low	B, G3+D	Lemon and Scarlet on Systemic Front and Systemic Back or Whole Body Front and Whole Body Back.
Cancer	B, D#	Lemon on Systemic Front, including Affected Area; Indigo on Affected Area.
Cigarette Smoking	C, A	Green on Systemic Front to repair damage; Orange and Lemon on Upper and Lower Chest.
Drug Addiction	C, G+E/G#+D	Green on Systemic Front; Magenta or Scarlet on Chest and Abdomen if heart rate is low.
Insomnia	E, A#+E	Violet on Crown of Head; Purple on Crown of Head, Throat and Chest
Insanity	C, G+E	Green on Crown of head and/or Systemic Front, then Magenta on Systemic Front.
Nervous Condition	B, A# B, A	Lemon and Yellow on Systemic Front and Systemic Back for 2 weeks; then Lemon and Orange on Systemic Front and Systemic Back for 4 weeks (may repeat once).
Stress, Seizures	E; A#+E	Violet on Crown of Head or Purple on Crown of Head, Throat, and Chest if pulse rate is high.
Stroke with Paralysis	A#+E, D# B, G+E	Purple on Crown of Head, Throat, and Chest and Indigo on Whole Body Front and Forehead; later use Lemon on Systemic Front; Magenta on Crown of Head, Throat, and Chest.

Systemic Front = Neck to Hips on front of body.

Systemic Back = Neck to Hips on back of body.

Whole Body Front = Top of Head to Bottoms of Feet on Front of Body.

Whole Body Back = Top of Head to Bottoms of Feet on Back of Body.

Affected Area = Organs or Parts of the Body that are experiencing symptoms.

Colored Lights are applied as directed. Tone is intermittent (2-3 minute duration with 7-8 minute pauses) and in the background, while the body is experiencing the light therapy.

Technique:

1. Do not eat or bathe one hour before filtered light treatment and toning therapy.
2. Set up 6 ounces of water in a glass to be exposed to the color combination desired for one hour.
3. Preheat room to 80° F. Set clock for 1 hour.
4. Prepare person for the filtered light treatment and toning therapy. Adjust as needed.
5. Darken room and allow person to absorb music and warmth for 5 minutes.
6. Allow person to drink color-treated water over 10 minutes.
7. Situate person for filtered light treatment and toning therapy for 40 minutes.
8. Darken room and allow person to relax without light for 5 minutes.
9. Do not eat or bathe for one hour after filtered light treatment and toning therapy.

PART TWO
CROSS REFERENCE GUIDE

HERB	AILMENTS
A	
Alfalfa	Indigestion, Ulcers
Aloe Vera	Burns, Bites, Rash
Anise	Bad Breath, Cough
Apple	Fever
B	
Basil	Lactation
Bay	Indigestion
Bearberry (Uva Ursi, Kinnickinnick)**	Astringent, Kidney Problems, Dizziness, Tinnitus, Vertigo
Beech	Ivy Poison, Oak Poison
Birch	Antiseptic, Boils, Diarrhea, Worms
Black Cohosh	Cramps, Sedative
Blueberry	Diabetes
Borage	Fever, High Blood Pressure, Kidney Problems, Laxative, Weakness
Burdock	Antiseptic, Burns, Boils, Flu, Hemorrhoids, Measles, Ringworm, Sores
C	
Cabbage	Rheumatism, Worms, Drawing, Dry Lactation
Calendula (Marigolds)	Acne, Inflammation, Rash, Scars, Sprains
Carrots	Sores, Worms
Cattail	Bandaging
Cayenne	Cramps, Sore Throat
Celery	Nerves
Chamomile	Allergies, Dyspepsia, Eczema, Nerves
Charcoal	Gangrene
Chickweed	Burns, Constipation
Chia Seeds	Endurance, Energy, Brain Function
Clover – Red	Boils, Cancer, Hot Flashes, Nerves, Vomiting
Clover – White	Boils, Cancer, Vomiting
Cloves	Toothache
Comfrey	Anemia, Antiseptic, Burns, Boils, Cough, Cuts, Diarrhea, Gangrene, Hemorrhage, Pneumonia, Rupture, Sprains
Corn Silk	Bed-wetting
Cranberry	Cystitis, Kidney Disorders
Cucumber	Prostate Cancer

HERB	AILMENTS
D	
Dandelion	Anemia, UTI, Diabetes, Skin Disease, Nerves, Pain
Dill	Nerves, Pain
Devil's Claw	Arthritis Pain
E	
Echinacea	Bronchitis, Colds, Flu, HIV
Eucalyptus	Stuffy nose, Stuffy sinuses
F	
Fennel	Gas, Gargle, Worms
Fungus, Tree	Antiseptic, Bandaging
G	
Garlic	Antiseptic, Colds, Diabetes, Encephalitis, Earache, Gargle, Hot Flashes, Sores, Wounds, Yeast Infection
Ginger	Arthritis, Colds, Constipation, Dyspepsia, Headache Motion Sickness, Nausea, Sore Throat, Vertigo
Gingko Biloba	Alzheimer's Disease, Dementia, Cerebral Circulation, Vertigo
Goldenrod	Cough, Chest Trouble, Pleurisy
Goldenseal	Cankers, Disinfectant, Diabetes, Gingivitis, Gargle, Heart Problems, Hemorrhoids, Infections, Ivy and Oak Poison, Laxative, Mouthwash, Tonsillitis, Yeast Infection, Vaginitis
H	
Hyssop	Cough, Pain
Hawthorn**	Dizziness, Anxiety, Tinnitus, Vertigo
Hibiscus Flowers** Hibiscus Leaves**	Liver support, Weight control, Diabetes, Menstrual Cramps, Depression, Laxative Pimples, Acne
I	
Indian Frankincense (Boswellia Extract)	Arthritis Pain and Swelling

HERB	AILMENTS
J	
Juniper**	Kidney Stones, Aches, Dizziness, Vertigo, Tinnitus
K	
Kinnickinnick With Dandeline root	Vaginal Wash UTI
L	
Lady's Slipper	Appendicitis
Lavender	Depression, Headache, Pain
Lemon	Itching, Earache
Licorice	Ulcers
Linseed Oil	Cough
Lobelia*	Boils, Fever, Nausea, Nerves, Vomiting
M	
Marigold (Calendula)	Acne, Inflammation, Rash, Scars, Sprains
Marshmallow	Coughs, Diuretic, Diabetes, Lactation, Pneumonia, Vaginal Wash, Tooth Cutting
Milkweed	Cirrhosis, Gallstones, Hepatitis, Warts
Mullein*	Sleep Inducer, Tumors, Warts
Medical Marijuana	Stress, Nervousness, Pain, Cancer Pain, Seizures, Brain Fog, Tremors, Dementia, TBI Symptoms affecting mobility and speech
N	
Nature-dried Pine Sap	Bandaging
Nettles	Colds, Hay Fever, Hemorrhage, Osteoporosis, Pain, Tumors, Worms
O	
Olive Leaves*	Pulmonary, CHF, Dizziness, Vertigo, Tinnitus

HERB	AILMENTS
P	
Parsley	Fever, Gallstones, Insect Bites
Peach	Constipation
Pennyroyal*	Convulsions, Fever, Headache, Insect Bites, Nausea, Skin Disease, Mouth Sores, Snake Bite, Toothache, Eczema
Peppermint	Aches, Colds, Convulsions, Colitis, Diverticulitis, Diarrhea, Flu, Gas, Heart Problems, Headache, Nausea, Sleep Inducer, Vomiting
Plantain	Antiseptic, Burns, Hemorrhage, Insect Bites, Pimples, Eczema, Sores, Swelling, Snake-Bite, Toothache, Wounds
Poplar	Aches, Fever, Flu, Gangrene, Headache, Worms, Weakness
Pumpkin	Prostate Cancer
Papaya Enzyme (Papain)	Arthritis Pain
Pineapple Enzyme (Bromelain)	Arthritis Pain and Swelling
Q	
R	
Raspberry	Anemia, Diuretic, Diabetes, Eczema
Rhubarb	Constipation, Gallstones, Headache
Rosemary	Alzheimer's Disease, Dementia, Cough, Headache
S	
Sage	Colds, Dandruff, Fever, Gas, Gargle, Inflammation, Laxative, Pneumonia, Worms, Cancer
Sassafras	Pneumonia, Worms, Cancer
Slippery Elm*	Boils
Solomon Seal	Wounds
Soy	Hot Flashes
Spearmint	Indigestion
St. John's Wort	Antiseptic, Burns, Cuts, Rash
Strawberry	Diarrhea, Gas
Summer Savory	Colds, Toothache

HERB	AILMENTS
T	
Tee Tree Oil	Antifungal, Athlete's Foot, Boils, Infection, Headlice
Thyme	Antiseptic, Cramps, Headache
Tree Fungus	Antiseptic, Bandaging
Turmeric	Arthritis
U	
Uva Ursi/Bearberry / Kinnickinnick*	Dizziness, Tinnitus, UTI or Kidney Infections
V	
Vervain	Appendicitis, Colds, Fever
W	
Watercress	Inflammation
White Pine	Flu
Willow	Anxiety, Arthritis, Pneumonia, Toothache
Wintergreen	Myalgia (Sore Muscles)
X	
Y	
Yarrow	Colds, Pleurisy, Hemorrhage, Measles, Toothache
Yellow Dock	Ringworm
Yucca	Arthritis Pain
Z	

*Be careful of the strength of the tea as it may cause deep, prolonged sleep.
**DO NOT give to pregnant women (may cause miscarriage).

PART THREE
GENERAL USES

Portion	Method	Application
Roots	Finely Cut	Boil ½ hour or more
Bark	Finely Cut	Boil ½ hour or more
Flowers	Cut	Simmer in a covered dish
Leaves	Cut	Simmer in a covered dish
	Bruised	Use fresh by direct application
Powder	In Water	½ teaspoon to 2 oz. water, followed by a full 8-ounces of water
Charcoal	Willow Coconut Shell Pine	1 heaping teaspoon added to enough water to make a paste, dilute and drink

SCENTS

HERB	PREPARATION
Lavender, Lilac, Carnations, Hibiscus	Sachets – dry blossoms, crush fine, place in cloth bags.
Roses	Rosewater – cover rose petals with water and boil. Cool and strain. Store in a glass jar out of direct sunlight. Use for oily skin. Sachets – dry blossoms, crush fine, place in cloth bags.
Lemon	Lemon Balm Perfume – cover lemon balm petals with water and boil. Cool and strain. Store in a glass jar out of direct sunlight. Use for dry skin.

USE OF "WATER-GLASS" TO KEEP EGGS FRESH WITHOUT REFRIGERATION

In the days before refrigeration or in areas without refrigeration, a substance called "water glass" was/is used to preserve eggs. This can be purchased from a pharmacy, although today you must explain why you want it. According to my own testing, the eggs may be preserved in the following way:

1. Use farm fresh eggs.
2. Wash the eggs very thoroughly as dirt may cause them to rot.
3. Candle the eggs to assure that you are using unfertilized eggs only. Fertilized eggs will rot.
4. Pack eggs in a bucket with a lid, but first, put down a layer of "water glass" (it will become like a gelatin).
5. As you pack each layer of eggs, cover completely with "water glass" and let it set until firm before adding another layer.
6. Because you may not have enough fresh eggs all at once, it may take you two or three weeks to fill the bucket with fresh eggs. Make sure each layer is well covered with no air pockets.
7. Leave a 4 inch head space at the top of the bucket in insure that all eggs are well covered with "water glass."
8. When a bucket is filled, add clean bubble wrap or crumpled paper for padding. Do not use newsprint as the ink will promote deterioration.
9. Put the lid on the bucket firmly, label with the date, then turn the bucket upside down to store.
10. Every three to six weeks, turn the bucket over. Label the bucket with the date of the last 'turn.'
11. Eggs should keep fresh for six months to a year when stored in a cool, dry place (40-60°).
12. As you use the eggs, be sure to use a complete layer at once time, not breaking the seal to lower layers.

HELPFUL HINTS

Uses for Peroxide

- Take one little capful and hold in your mouth for 10 minutes daily, then spit out. No more canker sores and your teeth will be whiter, too!

- After rinsing off your wooden cutting board or rolling pin, pour peroxide on it to kill salmonella and other bacteria.

- Soak any infections or cuts in 3% peroxide for 5-10 minutes, several times a day. Also works to clean gangrene.

- Add a cupful of peroxide instead of bleach to a load of whites and watch as even blood stains disappear!

- Lighten yellowed toenails by soaking them with peroxide.

- Gargle a capful to cure a newly acquired sore throat.

Uses for Salt

- Dissolve a teaspoonful of salt in a small glass of warm water. Gargle to cure a sore throat.

- Use dry salt on your hands to rid them of odors like onion and garlic.

- Lightly sprinkle salt on your shelves to repel ants.

- A tiny pinch of salt in egg whites makes them beat up fluffier.

- Add a little salt to warm milk to have a more relaxing drink.

- Salt water helps fruits to not discolor.

- Salt and lemon juice remove mildew.

Uses for Apple Cider Vinegar

- It's a cleaner! It shines almost anything. It isn't harmful to humans, animals, or the environment. Use it on glass, floors, metal, etc.

- It's helpful for diabetes. Added to your foods, it can help you maintain your blood sugar levels.

Uses for Baking Soda

- It's a cleaner! It disinfects and leaves no smell or residue. It doesn't shine like vinegar, but it helps destroy germs. It is especially good for cleaning the refrigerator or your animal's dishes.

- It will whiten your teeth. Make a paste out of baking soda and water, with a little salt, and brush the germs and stains away.

FUN STUFF

3P + C

For relief of most common ailments, remember:

Three P's and a C.

That is:
Peppermint
Plantain
Pennyroyal
And Comfrey

They help cure – flu, colds, nausea, vomiting, diarrhea, and headaches.

Peppermint Tea
= For cuts, burns, sores, inflammations, and swelling
Also upset stomach and cold/flu symptoms

Plantain Poultice or Wash
= For insect bites, bruises, rash, and fever

Pennyroyal Poultice
= For coughs, toothache, and eczema

Comfrey Tea or Fresh Application
= For antiseptic on cuts, burns and boils

Garlic has an age-old reputation as a plant that stirs sexual appetites and rambunctious thoughts. Be careful when using this herb!

THE WEED GATHERERS

Become familiar with a plant.
Make friends with a weed.
Herbs can make a difference,
And help in times of need.

Some trips into the forest,
Traipsing across the fields;
A bag full of treasures,
Our days of toiling yields.

Cleaning, cutting, drying herbs;
Putting knowledge to use.
Finding new recipes
For healing, foods, and juice.

Building up our yearly supply,
Preparing to meet our needs;
Finding friends and comfort
Inside a bunch of 'weeds.'
- S.T. 1987

SPICY PHARMACY

If a pain you want to still,
Try a little of your DILL.
But, if you've eaten too much for dinner,
Perhaps you'll want to try some GINGER!

GARLIC sure will clean a sore,
While THYME, headaches make 'no more.'
If beans have set your tummy a-rage,
Maybe you'd like to try some SAGE.

Juice of LEMON, for an itch.
CAYENNE capsules for a 'stitch.'
SUMMER SAVORY for colds is best,
CELERY seeds calm nerves, so you can rest.

Kidneys just love CUCUMBER,
PUMPKIN seeds will make them purr.
And BAY LEAVES can help indigestion,
While CLOVE OIL makes toothaches more fun!

For a fever, try PARSLEY.
And for a cough, ROSEMARY.
So, there on your shelf is, right at hand;
The best home pharmacy in the land.

▪ M.S.T., 1980

Uses:

Dill Seeds – Eat Raw	Sage Leaf – Tea, Drink	Celery Seeds – Eat, Raw	Clove Oil – Rub On
Ginger – Tea, Drink	Lemon Juice – Wash	Cucumber Seeds – Eat Raw	Parsley Leaf – Wash
Garlic – Poultice	Cayenne Cap – Take Orally	Pumpkin Seeds – Eat Raw	Bay Leaf – Tea Drink
Rosemary Leaf – Tea Drink	Thyme Leaf – Tea Drink	Summer Savory – Tea Drink	

Cancer treatment using natural herbs.

Make a strong tea from red clover blossoms. Drink daily.

For sores or "cancerous spots" on your skin, make a mild tea of sage roots and wash the area daily until it disappears (may take a few weeks, so have patience).

Eat cucumber seeds from fresh cucumbers daily as a preventative.

A mixture of blue violet leaves, burdock, yellow dock, dandelion root, and golden seal – make a tea and drink daily.

Slipper elm root, willow, poplar, poke root – simmer together into a tea, use as a poultice on affected skin spots.

Cancer Treatment:
Step One: Cleanse the body by using an herbal laxative (recipe below). Use a high enema of marshmallow tea. This may also be used as an effective douche.

Step Two: Eat fresh fruits of all kinds, including tomatoes, for the first 10 days to 2 weeks. Vegetable and unsweetened fruit juices are also recommended, plus water. Drink red clover blossom tea in place of water most of the time. Do not take your herb drink for at least one hour after drinking/eating vegetables and fruits. Do not eat fruits and vegetables at the same meal, or drink fruit and vegetable drinks at the same time. Allow them to work separately in your body for 1-2 hours.

Fruit List	Vegetable List	Herb List
Oranges	Celery	Red Clover Blossoms
Grapefruit	Green Lima Beans	Burdock Root
Lemons	Onions, Garlic	Yellow Dock Root
Apples	Wild Rice, Lentils	Blue Violet Plant
Cranberries	Cauliflower	Golden Seal Root
Unsweetened Blueberries	Potatoes, Baked	Gum Myrrh
Red Raspberries	Yellow Corn Meal	Echinacea
Cherries	Cucumbers	Aloe
Peaches	Fresh Garden Lettuce	Bloodroot
Pears	Radishes, Beets	Dandelion Root

Ripe Strawberries
Avocados
Pineapple
Tomatoes
Watermelon
Rhubarb Root
Chinese Cabbage

Watercress
Spinach
Squash
Kale and Swiss Chard
Asparagus
Dandelion Greens
Sage
Wheat, Soy Bean Sprouts

Chickweed
Oregon Grape
Irish Ivy
Marshmallow Leaves
Hyssop
Mullein

Cancer treatment using natural herbs, continued.

Both watermelon and tomatoes should be eaten alone, not with any other fruit or vegetables due to the lycopene content.

Step Three: Get plenty of fresh air and exercise, soak up as much sunshine as possible. Use deep breathing exercises as well as low impact exercises for the entire body.

Step Four: Soak in hot water daily, followed by a salt water rinse. This will help purify the skin. Remember to use a cool rinse after the salt water to clean off excess salt.

Step Five: Alternate hot and cold applications to the liver, stomach, spleen, and spine, especially after the soaking treatment in step four. Simply apply a hot or cold compress to each area, alternating them, over about a 10-minute time span, daily.

Step Six: Burn either sage or sweetgrass in an incense burner to purify the air in your home or room, daily. Alternate the two, one on one day and the other on the next day.

Step Seven: Mix together, golden seal, hyssop, mullein, rhubarb, sage, Oregon grape, and aloe and steep into a tea. Use 1/4th teaspoon mixture to a 4-ounce cup of warm water. Follow with a glass of plain, warm water. This mixture can also be used as an enema if the case is rectal and severe, or as a douche if the case is vaginal and severe.

Repeat this process as long as necessary for your personal case.

Medical Marijuana has also been found to ease pain and anxiety associated with cancer.

Liver Treatment:

1. Drink a mixture of Fennel, Parsley, Plantain, and Aloe. Eat Carrots, Celery, and Dandelion Blossoms. This is a daily treatment.
2. Golden Seal, Lobelia, Milkweed, Rhubarb, Sage, and Poke Root. Take daily as a mild tea, in small amounts (2 ounces), followed by warm water.

Diet for Diabetes

For the first three weeks, eat lean meat and salad with lite dressing only. Water only to drink.

No pasta, no potatoes, no bacon bits, no croutons, beans or fruit for the first three weeks.

No cereals or breads for the first three weeks.

Salad may contain egg and a small amount of cheese.

After you go through the first three weeks, you should see a beginning of weight loss.

You may then eat one small helping of potatoes per week, two helpings of pasta per week, and two to three helpings of fruit per week. You may also resume eating white rice three to four times per week.

NO DESSERTS FOR TWO MONTHS! NO SODA OF ANY KIND! NO FRUIT JUICES FOR TWO MONTHS!

Remember to keep servings small and do not have seconds.

After you get down to your target weight (or close), you may add desserts once a week, and once in a while, have a second small helping of a favorite entrée. When you have bread again, use only whole grain breads, or a true French or Italian loaf.

You may eat a small amount of oatmeal or creamy wheat once a week. You may have fruit juice occasionally.

Make it a life commitment, you are changing your way of eating forever, not just to lose weight temporarily.

Diet for Arthritis

This is a modification of your normal diet.

It is a low carb and sugar diet.

Do not eat bagels, muffins, or breads more than twice per week.

Do not eat blackened or barbecued foods.

Do not eat processed foods, French fries, use soya oil or eat peanuts.

Limit your use of beets and root vegetables such as carrots or potatoes.

Limit your sugars to one time per week.

To sweeten tea or coffee, use honey instead of sugar.

Do not eat white rice.

You may eat citrus fruits in moderation.

You may eat fruit, fresh vegetables, and lean meats. Limit your red meat intake.

Coffee, soda, and fruit juices should be eliminated from your diet.

PART FOUR
PREPARATIONS

Preparation	Application
Powdered Herbs	½ teaspoonful to ¼ of a 6-ounce glass of water, followed by a 6-ounce glassful of very warm water.
Syrups	Honey and cut herb boiled into a syrup, strained through a double layer of cheesecloth, then bottled. 2 ounces of dried herb (4 ounces fresh) to 1 quart water, boil down to 1 pint and add 2 ounces of honey. Bottle to use as needed.
Salves	Cut fresh herbs finely, 1 pound of herb to 1 ½ pounds of cocoa fat (or olive, sunflower, almond, or sesame oils) and 4 ounces of beeswax. Mix well, and cover, leaving in the hot sun for 13-14 hours. Strain through a fine cloth, mix well until it is smoothed and creamed together. Cool and store in a sealed jar or container. (If using an oven, it takes about 2-3 hours. If using a microwave, it takes about 20 minutes).
Poultices	Use ground herbs made into a paste using water. Spread paste on cheesecloth and wrap firmly. Wash affected area with peroxide, then apply the poultice. Cover tightly with towels and/or sheeting. Change hourly so as not to burn the skin.
Infusion	Bruise plant leaves and steep in one quart of just-boiled water for about 15 minutes. The liquid may be used internally or externally. About 1 pint of water to 2 cups of dried herb or 4 cups of fresh herb.
Tincture	Use one or two ounces of powdered herb to one quart of alcohol. Let stand for two weeks before use. Store in a colored glass container in a dark, cool place. External use only.

Preparation	Application
Essences	One to two ounces of oil from the desired herb to one quart of alcohol. Let stand two weeks before use. Store in a colored glass container in a dark, cool place. External use only.
Decoction	Boil water and add herb. Keep simmering just under boiling for ½ hour. One pint water to 2 cups dried herb or 4 cups fresh herb. 1 teaspoon for a child or the elderly, 2 teaspoons for a teen, 1 Tablespoon for an adult. Every six hours as needed.
Liniment	Wash or rub for affected parts. See Recipes
Laxative	¼ teaspoon put into ¼ 6-ounce glass of cold water, followed by a 6-ounce glassful of very warm water.
Tonic	½ teaspoonful dried herb in ¼ 8-ounce glass of cold water, followed by a 8-ounce glassful of very warm water.
Herb Oil	2 ounces of dried herbs or 4 ounces of fresh herbs, ground finely. Add 1 pint of olive oil (almond, sunflower, or sesame oils). Mix well and stand in the sun for 3 days, or simmer over wood heat for 5-6 hours, or heat in oven on low for 4-5 hours, or heat in a microwave for 25 minutes. Strain and bottle the oil. Store in a dark, cool place.
Ointment	Cover the finely ground herb with olive oil (almond, sunflower, or sesame oil) in a glass jar. Place in the sun for 21 days. Strain and store ointment in a glass container in a cool, dark place.

Preparation	Application
Lard Salve	Bring 2# of pork or bear lard to the point of smoking heat. Add finely cut herb (about ¼ pound) and mix well. Coo. Reheat to 'popping heat' stage. Cool enough to strain through cheesecloth. Let the liquid set one week in a lightly covered container before sealing. Keep cool.
Fomentation	Warm, moist compress. Usually moistened with herbal tea.
Capsules	Using a commercial gel-cap, fill with powdered herb. Be sure of the individual dose for each capsule, usually ¼ to ½ teaspoon of powder to one capsule.
Paste	Use powdered herb with enough pure olive oil or water to make it into a pasty substance. Most pastes may be applied directly to the skin, unless the herb or vegetable is high in acidity and needs to be used in a poultice form or wrapped in damp cloth to keep the substance from affecting the skin.
Distilled Oil	Use fresh herb leaves and flowers, chopped. Add to about a ½ crockpot full of distilled water. Heat on high until steaming, Turn to low and simmer for about 3 hours. Put the pot into the fridge overnight. Carefully skim the oil off the top of the water. Store oil in a colored bottle, in a dark, cool, dry place.

FRUITS & VEGETABLES, MEAT & WATER – BENEFITS, AND ABOUT EATING THEM
(See nutrition tables elsewhere in this book)

It is best to eat vegetables raw or steamed. When you cook foods, it causes a breakdown of their nutritive value. Steamed vegetables still contain their nutrients and are softened for easy chewing and digestion. Almost all vegetables contain Vitamin A and many greens contain high amounts of Vitamin K. some are higher in Potassium than others. Potatoes have long since been regarded as a complete food when eaten with their skins on. Carrots are known for their high content of Vitamin A. Legumes should be eaten sparingly. However, they do contain a high value of protein.

Fruits should always be eaten raw and on an empty stomach. They cushion the acids in the stomach for any other foods you might eat and clean out your digestive system when eaten regularly. Tomatoes are high in Lycopene, an antioxidant for healthy bodies. Fruits may prevent many fatal diseases, including cancers. A fruit and fruit juice cleanse once or twice a year is recommended for total health.

Meat is meant to be eaten. It is more harmful to not eat white or 'lighter' meats in the spring and summer, and to eat it sparingly so as not to overload your digestive system. Red or 'heavy' meats are best to be eaten in the fall and winter, when your body needs extra warmth and fats to burn. Again, eat sparingly. Two to four ounces of meat for a meal is enough to satisfy and to remain healthy.

A few words about chocolate (cocoa):
Chocolate is promoted highly. It tastes wonderful and makes one "feel good." The health benefits are not so great. Cocoa is a filler of sorts, contains 1% simple sugar, and is 50% fat, making it cling to cells. Cocoa goes into your cells and takes up space while more healthful foods are sloughed off, their nutrients cast out of your system because they can't be used. Chocolate also contains polyphenols similar to those found in wine, throbromine, a mild stimulant, and natural caffeine, also found in kola tree nuts and in tea leaves. Cocoa takes time to be absorbed (even up to 5-10 days depending on your metabolism and habits), so weigh carefully the

taste against the benefits (or lack thereof) to your body. Drinking lots of water will help shorten the time it takes for cocoa to be absorbed in your body. Citrus juices or fruits ingested when eating cocoa products also help your body to digest cocoa more readily. Cocoa is toxic to dogs, cats, parrots, and horses causing their bodily functions to clog up and threatening their lives. It has been said to cause human bodies to produce extra amounts of serotonin, making one feel calm and serene while it rids your body of nutrition.

About drinking water and other drinks:
Water should be drunk at room temperature. Iced water and drinks cause foods to congeal and slow down the bodily digestive processes along with the nutritive value of the foods you eat. Hot water and drinks cause reactions in the stomach (besides getting your tongue burned in the process), which are not beneficial to the normal breakdown of foods to be used by your waiting cells. Healing teas should be used tepid to cool, never hot or cold.

Testing toxicity in wild mushrooms:
Place the fungus in a glass bowl filled with cold water and 2 Tablespoons salt. If water turns a bright orange, blue, or green, the mushrooms cannot be eaten. Water may turn brown-looking from the fungus itself, but that is a natural color. The mushrooms may be eaten.

Nutrition Information:
Potassium keeps a healthy water balance between your cells and body fluids.

Calcium eases insomnia and promotes healthy bones and teeth.

Iron and Vitamin C work together to strengthen your body systems.

Iron works to neutralize the effects of Vitamin E. Iron loss affects behavior and impairs learning abilities. It also lowers your immune system and causes fatigue and weakness.

Phosphorus is essential in fortifying blood cells and building bone structure. It is also connected to memory and synapse connectivity.

Magnesium is essential for maintenance of muscle mass and synapse connectivity for nervous tension. It boots immunity and blood pressure regulation.

Tobacco leaf wraps are good for treating bruises and sprains in cattle, horses, goats, sheep, pigs, and llamas.

Tannin in Pekoe Teas cause the body to slough off precious amounts of iron. Tannin may create a depletion of blood cell productivity and liver malfunction.

Caffeine causes irregularities in synapse connectivity and interrupts sleep patterns. It has been shown to be related to dementia and tremors. Caffeine is found in cocoa plants, coffee beans, and teas naturally.

Nicotine creates a tar that builds up in lungs and airways. It also creates irregularities in synapse connectivity and interrupts natural emotional ease. It has been related to the production of active cancer cells in the body as well as producing dangerous blood clots. Nicotine is found in tobacco plants.

Distilled spirits (whiskey, rum, vodka, etc.) create synapse irregularities and memory fatigue. It can cause memory loss or interruptions and break down enzymes needed to process foods for nutritive value, including erosion in the liver and other vital digestive organs.

Vitamins:

A	Protects against measles. Promotes cell reproduction. Promotes a healthy immune system. Good for vision, bones teeth, skin, hair, and mucous membranes. Found in liver, fish, carrots, broccoli, cantaloupe, and squash.
B-1 Thiamine	Converts carbs into energy. Promotes healthy heart function, muscles, and nervous system. Found in yeast, beans, liver, nuts, oats, oranges, eggs, pork, and peas.
B-2	Promotes body growth and red cell reproduction. Found in milk, cheese, eggs, beef, liver, chicken breast, and salmon.
B-3 Niacin	Promotes good cholesterol and lowers bad cholesterol when taken in modest amounts. Found in yeast, mushrooms, peanuts, tuna and salmon, chicken breast, and beef liver.

B-6	Promotes antibodies in the immune system. Causes the proper chemical reaction of proteins in the body. Lack causes dizziness, nausea, confusion, irritability, and convulsions. Found in pork, poultry, peanuts, wheat germ, oats, and bananas.
B-9	Promotes DNA health and brain function. Found in beans, peanuts, sunflower seeds, fruit, cereal grains, liver, and seafood.
B-12	Promotes a healthy metabolism and red cell reproduction. It is also essential in memory function. Found in liver, clams, tuna, trout, salmon, crab, eggs, milk, and cheese.
Complex	Promotes overall health to body and cognitive function. Found in milk, cheese, eggs, liver, meats, fish, spinach, and kale.
C	Greatest antioxidant and antiviral. Protects against heart and pulmonary disorders and cancer. Found in citrus fruits, peppers, berries, broccoli, brussels sprouts, and potatoes.
D	Aids the body in absorption of all other nutrients. Gotten primarily from the sun, 10 to 15 minutes, 3 times a week is sufficient for normal body function. Found in tuna, salmon, mushrooms, egg yolks, and red meats.
D-3	Aids in the absorption of calcium and phosphorus and to prevent osteoporosis. Found in salmon, tuna, beef liver, egg yolks, and cheeses.
E	Another, if lesser, antioxidant, aiding in the production of red blood cells. Also good to heal and soothe skin cells, reducing the effect of scarring. Without the effects of iron, it may generate over-production and cause metabolism damage. Found in sunflower and soy oils, almonds, peanuts, beet and collard greens, spinach, pumpkin, and red bell peppers.
K	Promotes blood clotting and bone health. Found in green leafy vegetables, broccoli, brussels sprouts, cabbage, fish, eggs, liver, and cereal grains.

Flavonoids	Antioxidants. Reduce the oxidization in cells which leads to major diseases including cancer. Promotes and supports eye, bone, and skin health. Found in dark chocolate, red cabbage, onions, kale, parsley, berries, peaches, and tomatoes.
Phosphorus	Aids in building red blood cells (anorexia, anemia), proximal muscle weakness, bone pain, risk of infection and mental confusion. Found in vegetables, fruits, whole grain, low-fat milk, fish, nuts and beans.
Magnesium	Supports muscle and nerve function, blood pressure regulation, and the immune system. Found in nuts, dark chocolate, avocados, legumes, chia, whole grains, salmon, bananas, spinach, kale, and pumpkin seeds.

PART FIVE

RECIPES

NOTE: Check all equipment used to make sure no copper or
iron from un-plated spoons, colanders, shredders, chipped enamel
vessels, or other utensils comes in contact with the product.
If it does, Vitamin C is instantly destroyed.
<u>NEVER USE ALUMINUM UTENSILS OR PANS!</u> USE GLASS ONLY!

Soap:

Soapwort	Beat roots in water until sudsy.
Yucca	Beat roots in water until sudsy.
Making Lye:	Bring hardwood ashes to a boil.
	Cool and strain – liquid will be your lye.

Making lye soap:
One gallon of lye to 5 gallons of soft water and 9 pounds of grease.
Add ½ pound of borax.
Boil about 2 hours or until the grease floats and is soapy.
Add ½ pound of salt and boil another ½ hour.
Soak a tub in cold water and pour the soap in to cool.
Let the soap stand until it is cold.
Cut soap into cakes or flake it for use in washing clothes.

Toothpaste:
4 Tablespoons baking soda
6 Tablespoons coconut oil
20-25 drops of essential oils (grapefruit, eucalyptus, peppermint, spearmint, etc.)
1 teaspoon Stevia or other sweetener
Store in a small, covered container.

Salves:

Balm of Gilead, Comfrey, or Plantain (for cuts and wounds):
4-5 pounds of herb leaves barely covered with goose, bear, or pork grease.
Simmer 5-6 hours (40-50 minutes in the microwave)
Add a few bees wax shavings.
Cool slightly and strain into glass jars.
Let the salve set lightly covered until solid.
Store in a cool, dry place.

Chickweed or Calendula (Marigold) (for rashes and chapped skin or lips):
>2 ½ pounds of herb leaves, finely ground
>Cut into 1 ½ pounds cocoa butter or,
>2 cups pure oil (olive, sunflower, sesame, or almond)
>Add 10 ounces bees wax
>Mix and cover
>Set in hot sun or in oven on low heat for 3-4 hours or,
>20 minutes in the microwave
>Cool and strain into glass jars
>Let it set until solid
>Store in cool, dry place

Burdock or St. John's Wort (for burns and boils):
>1 pound of leaves and stems of the herb
>1 ½ pounds cocoa butter or
>2 cups pure oil (olive, sunflower, sesame, or almond)
>4 ½ ounces bees wax
>Set in hot sun or in oven on low heat for 3-4 hours or,
>20 minutes in microwave
>Cool and strain into glass jars
>Let it set until solid
>Store in cool, dry place

Hibiscus (for depression):
>1 pound of flowers and berries of the herb
>1 ½ pounds cocoa butter or
>2 cups pure oil (olive, sunflower, sesame, or almond)
>4 ½ ounces bees wax
>Set in hot sun or in oven on low heat for 3-4 hours or,
>20 minutes in microwave
>Cool and strain into glass jars
>Let it set until solid
>Store in cool, dry place
>Rub on bottoms of feet at night or when lying down

Hawthorn (for hyperactivity, anxiety):

> 1 pound of leaves and stems of the herb
> 1 ½ pounds cocoa butter or
> 2 cups pure oil (olive, sunflower, sesame, or almond)
> 4 ½ ounces bees wax
> Set in hot sun or in oven on low heat for 3-4 hours or,
> 20 minutes in microwave
> Cool and strain into glass jars
> Let it set until solid
> Store in cool, dry place
> Rub on bottoms of feet at night or when lying down

Drawing Salve:

> ½ cup sweet oil (olive)
> ½ cup bees wax
> ½ cup sheep fat
> ½ cup pork or bear leaf lard (from the loin or around kidneys, very soft)
> Heat each of these ingredients separately, then combine and boil together 10 minutes
> Add 1 Tablespoon unheated Turpentine and 3 drops Carbolic Acid
> Used to draw poison and infection from a wound by poultice.
> Hal Berger – Leavenworth, WA, circa 1900

Liniments:

For Pain:

> Mix well:
> 2 Tablespoons dried Comfrey
> 2 Tablespoons dried Yarrow
> 2 Tablespoons dried St. John's Wort
> Add 1 cup alcohol in a glass jar
> Seal and steep for 2 months, shake daily
> Turn jar weekly
> Strain and add 3-5 drops Peppermint Oil
> Bottle and store in cool, dark place
> Use as a rub.

For Arthritis:

Mix well: 2 Tablespoons dried Willow Bark
2 Tablespoons dried Yarrow
2 Tablespoons dried Cayenne
Add 1 cup alcohol in a glass jar
Seal and steep for 2 months, shake daily
Turn jar weekly
Strain and add 3-5 drops Peppermint Oil
Bottle and store in cool, dark place
Use as a rub.

For Bruises:

Mix well: 2 Tablespoons dried Arnica
2 Tablespoons dried Chamomile
2 Tablespoons dried Frankincense
Add 1 cup alcohol in a glass jar
Seal and steep for 2 months, shake daily
Turn jar weekly
Strain and add 3-5 drops Peppermint Oil
Bottle and store in cool, dark place
Use as a rub.

For Cramps:

Mix well: 2 Tablespoons dried Basil
2 Tablespoons dried Juniper
2 Tablespoons dried Myrrh
Add 1 cup alcohol in a glass jar
Seal and steep for 2 months, shake daily
Turn jar weekly
Strain and add 3-5 drops Peppermint Oil
Bottle and store in cool, dark place
Use as a rub.

Fever Drawing Poultice:

> Make a poultice of stewed pumpkins.
> Apply to boils and inflammations
> Renew every 15 minutes until fever is reduced.
> Then apply a good, mild liniment.
> American Agriculturist, circa 1900

Boil / Tumor Poultice:

> Make a poultice of roasted onions.
> Apply to boils, tumors, etc.
> Hastens suppuration.
> Often applied as 'drafts' to the feet.
> Change the poultice often until the boil or sore has 'drawn off'
> Circa, 1850

Sunburn Lotion:

> ½ ounce each: Dry beech leaves
>   Dry borage leaves
>   Dry comfrey leaves
>   Dry birch leaves
> Add: 1 pint alcohol
> Stir well.
> Let stand in glass jar, covered, for 7 days, stirring daily.
> Strain.
> Blend liquid with 1 cup aloe gel and 1 Tablespoon almond oil.
> Store in refrigerator.
> Shake well before use.
> Good for one season only. Discard any unused lotion.

Insect Repellant:

½ ounce each: Pennyroyal leaves
Eucalyptus leaves
Calendula (Marigold) leaves
Lavender leaves
Add: 2 cups alcohol
Stand in a glass jar, covered for 7 days, turning daily
Strain and discard leaves.
Date and label liquid. Use in a spray bottle. Good for one season only.

Bath Additive for Aches:

Mix: 1 ounce Burdock root
1 ounce Poplar bark
1 ounce Comfrey leaves
1 ounce Sage leaves
Add: 1 quart just-boiled water.
Steep for 10 minutes and strain
Add to bath.

Yeast Infection Treatment:

Mix: 1 ounce Marshmallow leaves
1 ounce Strawberry blossoms
Add to just-boiled water.
Steep for 10 minutes and strain.
Use as a wash and/or douche twice daily for 3 days.
Follow with:

Add strawberry leaves to just-boiled water
Steep for 10 minutes and strain.
Use as a wash and/or douche twice a day for 2 days.

UTI Treatment:

> Mix equal parts Kinnickinnick (Uva Ursi / Bearberry) leaves with
>
> Dandelion root.
>
> Add to just-boiled water.
>
> Steep for 5 minutes and strain.
>
> Drink twice daily.
>
> May also be used as a wash.

Laxative:

> Steep a very dark tea from Hibiscus Flowers.
>
> Drink one cup 3 times the first day.
>
> Drink one cup 2 times the second day.
>
> If the remedy is not working, consult your physician.

Cough Syrup:

> Boil juice of 1 lemon 10 minutes
>
> Mix with 1 cup honey
>
> Stir thoroughly before using

Cough and Cold Syrup:

> Mix well: 2 ounces dried comfrey leaves (4 ounces fresh)
>
> 1 ounce dried mullein leaves (2 ounces fresh)
>
> 1 ounce dried marshmallow leaves and stems (2 ounces fresh)
>
> Add: 2 quarts water
>
> Boil down to 2 pints.
>
> Add: 4 ounces honey
>
> Cool and strain
>
> Store in dark glass or closed cupboard.
>
> 1 teaspoonful every 4 hours as needed

Congestion:

Mix well: 2 ounces dried comfrey leaves (4 ounces fresh)

1 ounce dried mullein leaves (2 ounces fresh)

1 ounce dried marshmallow leaves and stems (2 ounces fresh)

½ ounce dried lobelia leaves (1 ounce fresh)

Store dry in a cool, dry place, well-sealed.

Make a VERY MILD tea and drink (about 2 teaspoonful to a 16 ounce pot of hot water.)

Brain Function Remedy:

1 cup dried Hawthorn Berries and Leaves

½ cup dried Juniper Berries

1 cup dried Rose Hips (Vitamin C)

1 cup Whole Egg Powder (Vitamin B12)

1 cup Potato Flour (Vitamin B6)

1 cup Yeast Powder (Vitamin B3)

¾ cup dried Hibiscus Flowers

1 cup dried Kinnickinnick Leaves (Bearberry; Uva Ursi)

1 cup dried Olive Leaves

Dried, crushed to powder, mixed well, and put into capsules.
1 capsule 2 times per day.

Dried, flaked, mixed well, and put into porous tea bags.
1 cup of tea, with honey, 2 times per day.

Boosts brain function.
Reduces headaches, tinnitus, and vertigo.
Moderates Non-epileptic seizure (NES) activity.
Renews synapse connectivity.
Supports overall bodily functions, pulmonary system, and the immune system.

THIS IS NOT FOR EPILEPSY! DO NOT USE THIS REMEDY IF YOU ARE PREGNANT OR NURSING!

Pectin:

Mix: 4 pounds sliced apples (peeled and cored)
4 pints water
Boil sliced apples for 20 minutes in a covered pot (NO aluminum)
Allow apples to drip through cheesecloth or a jelly bag without pressure
Save the liquid and return to pot
Heat until it cooks down to half its original volume
Store in sterilized glass jars or seal and process 15 minutes in boiling water baath

Rose Hip Extract (Vitamin C):

Gather rose hips and store in refrigerator until well chilled.
Wash quickly and remove stems and blossom ends.
Bring to a rolling boil in a glass pan.
1 ½ cup water for each cup of prepared rose hips.
Add:
1 cup chopped or mashed hips.
Cover with vapor-sealed lid.
Simmer 15 minutes.
Bring extract to a rolling boil again.
Add:
2 Tablespoons lemon juice per pint of liquid.
Pour into sterilized glass jars.
Seal for 15 minutes in boiling water bath

Dandelion Spread:

Combine: 1 cup young dandelion leaves
½ cup cottage cheese
½ cup chopped, ground nuts
Mix until smooth.
Add: homemade mayonnaise or
½ cup sour crème and ½ cup cream cheese
Add the mayonnaise to make the spread easy to smear over bread or crackers.

Yarrow Vinegar:

To ½ cup vinegar, add 5 or more young yarrow leaves (3-4 inches long)

Blend until leaves are finely chopped.

Let leaves settle, then taste the vinegar.

Add more leaves (1 at a time) for a stronger taste

Use in salad dressings

Birch Beer:

Finely cut 4 quarts birch twigs or inner bark, wash well

Add to 4 gallons water and about 1 cup birch sap (if available)

Bring to a full boil and add ½ to one gallon honey

Remove from heat and strain, discarding twigs and debris

Float 1 cake soft yeast on a piece of toast in liquid

Cover and let set for one week

Bottle and drink as desired.

Sassafras Tea:

Finely cut 4 quarts sassafras roots and inner bark, wash well

Add to 4 gallons water and ¼ teaspoon salt

Bring to a full boil and add 1 pint to 1 quart honey

Remove from heat and strain, discarding twigs and debris

Keep in refrigerator and drink as desired.

How to make Maple Syrup:

Choose your trees. Buy spiles to tap the trees.

Drill a hole about 2 inches into the tree, belt or chest high, slanting slightly up.

Tap the spile into the hole and hang a bucket on the spile.

Trees may produce ½ gallon to 5 gallons daily, depending on the temperature.

Collect syrup until you have enough to begin the boiling (about 10 gallons).

Boil on a burner outside so the steam doesn't deposit stickiness everywhere.

It takes about 40 gallons of sap to make around 1 gallon of syrup.

Boil it until it becomes thick and sweet, to about 219° F.

As the syrup heats, it will take on a brown hue.

Pour the syrup into glass jars and seal by using a boiling water bath for 15 minutes.

Store in a cool, dry place.

Electrolyte Solution:

¼ teaspoon salt

¼ teaspoon "no salt" (potassium chloride) *found in seasoning section of store

¼ teaspoon baking soda

2 ½ teaspoon sugar

Mix in 1 quart (four cups) water

You can also add 1/8 teaspoon Koolaid mix and 1 Tablespoon sugar for taste

Drink as much solution as possible during an episode of dehydration and sip it thereafter. This solution can be administered by enema in the case of vomiting (less the Koolaid and extra sugar).

PART SIX
SURVIVAL AND SAFETY

WATER STORAGE AND STERILIZATION

To Store and Use Tap Water:

2-liter, plastic pop bottles work best. Wash them out well then use bleach to rinse the bottles out, one more time. Rinse with water until the suds is no longer evident. Fill the bottles with cold water and seal. Date and rotate bottles every 10-12 months.

Some contaminants are chlorine-resistant. Good sand filtration will remove giardia. Boiling will destroy it. Giardia parasites are found in lakes, ponds, rivers and streams worldwide, as well as in public water supplies, wells, cisterns, swimming pools, water parks and spas.

To Disinfect Water of Unknown Potability:

1. Boiling – Filter the water though coffee filters, sand, or cheesecloth to remove any debris. Boil the water for 5-10 minutes to destroy any giardia. Let the water cool and settle. Use only the top ¾ of the water to avoid any small particulates. Treat with bleach (3 drops to 2 liters). The bleach kills disease-causing microorganisms. Shake water vigorously before drinking to improve the flavor.

2. Iodine – Do not use this method for lake or river water as it may not kill all microorganisms. Add 5 drops iodine tincture to 1 quart or 1 liter of water, or if the water is cloudy, add 10 drops. Let it stand for at least 30 minutes before using.

3. Chlorination - Treat with bleach (3 drops to 2 liters). The bleach kills disease-causing microorganisms. Shake water vigorously before drinking to improve the flavor.

4. Distillation – a) Use a commercial distiller; b) Build a distiller from plastic and place in a hole in the ground. Funnel water onto the plastic covering, allowing it to drip slowly through your filter into the container in the bottom. The water will still need to be treated with chlorine as above.

Plastic is the best material to use for the lining and covering of the distiller, and the holding box. The hole should be about 3 feet deep at the center. The box should be about 1 foot square. The filter should extend down about 1 ½ - 2 feet with a stone/pebble fitted to the hole to filter the water as it drips into the box. Surgical tubing will be used to draw up the water for use. Use rocks or blocks to hold the plastic and tubing in place.

5. Using water purifiers – pre-filter your water through a coffee filter, cheesecloth, or sand. Use commercial purifiers. However, the water will still need to be chlorinated.

6. Carbon filters – must be used for flood water or water that has been exposed to radiation. Water does not become radioactive and can be used after being run through a carbon filter.

SAFETY

Tips for EARTHQUAKE safety:
1. Go outside. Do not stay inside unless you have no other choice. Stay near the outer walls of a building.
2. Do not stay inside of a car. A natural void will most likely be formed beside the vehicle during an earthquake. Lie down beside your car.
3. Never go to stairs. Stairs are unstable during an earthquake and will grind and/or crush you.
4. Do not stand or sit in a doorway. The doorway will be one of the first things to be destroyed, and take you with it.
5. If you are in a motel room or cannot get out of your house, lie down in the fetal position at the foot of the bed or near a sofa or other bulky furniture item. A natural void will likely be formed beside these items of furniture during an earthquake.
6. Do not get under desks or vehicles, you will most likely be crushed.
7. Wooden buildings are the safest because they are more flexible. If they do collapse, they create large voids where you may survive.

Tips for TORNADO safety:
1. Practice tornado drills and be sure to teach your family about tornadoes and safety.
2. Be prepared with a emergency plan and access to a safe shelter. Safe shelters may be in basements, or a main floor room without windows. Wrap yourself in a blanket or a sleeping bag and cover your head with something soft and protective.

3. Avoid windows and get under something bulky and sturdy.
4. Never stay in a mobile home.
5. Keep an emergency kit with first aid supplies, 3-day supply of food and water, and batteries for an emergency radio.
6. Stay aware of the weather. Thunderstorms are indicative of tornado weather. Watch for hail, dark, low and swift moving clouds, a green tinge to the sky, or a roar like a train are indicators of tornadoes.

Tips for HURRICANE safety:
1. Crate a hurricane safety plan.
2. Know your evacuation route, 20-50 miles inland from the affected area.
3. Stock up on disaster supplies.
    a. Flashlights with extra batteries
    b. First aid kits, including an emotional first aid kit
    c. At least 72 hours of emergency food and water
    d. Essential medications and health supplies
    e. Non-electric can opener
    f. Local maps
4. Prepare your home/building. Check your local preparation requirements.
5. Drink plenty of water, eat well, wear sturdy work boots and wear gloves, wash your hands thoroughly with soap and clean water often when working with, in, and around debris.
6. Beware of new safety issues; washed out roads, contaminated buildings, contaminated water, gas leaks, broken glass, mold, damaged electrical wiring, slippery floors.
7. Inform local authorities about health and safety issues you observe.

Tips for FLOOD safety:
1. Find safe shelter right away.
2. Do not walk, swim, or drive through flood waters. Only one foot of flood water can sweep your vehicle away.
3. Stay off of bridges over swift-moving water.
4. Evacuate if told to do so.
5. Move to higher ground or a higher floor, even the roof, if necessary.
6. Stay where you are. Someone will find you.
7. Make a flood plan for yourself, your family, your pets or farm animals.

8. Build a 72-hour emergency kit with food, water, medicines, dry socks, and basic tools.
9. Know types of flood risk in your area.

Tips for WILDFIRE safety:
1. Secure your property before a wildfire happens:
   a. Within 30 feet of your home:
      Clear twigs, leaves, and pine needles
      Cut out dead limbs from existing trees
      Remove vines from the sides of your buildings
      Put away any flammable furniture when not in use
      Use stone or gravel instead of wood chips for décor
   b. Within 100 to 30 feet of your home:
      Create gravel or cement "fuel breaks"
      Cut tree branches that are within 8 feet from the ground
      Clear combustible vegetation (brambles, bushes, weeds)
   c. Within 200 to 100 feet from your home:
      Place any stacked firewood or scrap wood with care and consideration about fire
      Continue to clear combustible vegetation
      Plant trees far enough apart so their branches do not touch
2. Use Class A roofing on all your buildings.
3. Have sufficient garden hose to reach your entire property around your home.
4. Create an emergency escape plan.
5. Be prepared to evacuate quickly with a 72-hour emergency kit.
6. Move furniture to the center of your rooms. Take down drapes and curtains. Close all windows and doors. Shut off gas. Turn on all lights so firefighters can see your home through the smoke.
7. Return only when it is safe. Listen to authorities.
8. Be aware of ash pits that may still contain burning materials.

Tips for HOME INVASION safety:
1. Call 9-1-1.
2. Develop a code word that will tell your entire family that its time to spring into action.
3. Designate a "safe room" to gather together.

4. Do not leave the "safe room" for ANY reason.

5. If you are using a firearm for home defense, develop a "fatal funnel". Position yourself in a corner of the "safe room" with your family behind you, opposite the door. This will give you the maximum amount of safety and defensive advantage.

6. Stay in the "safe room" until the police arrive. They will find you.

Staying safe before a home invasion:

- Do not seek out or initiate a confrontation with an intruder.
- Get as far away from the intruder as possible.
- Call for help.
- Defend yourself if necessary,
- Have a plan and follow it.
- Don't make it obvious when you are home alone.
- Make sure your home is as secure as possible, door and window locks, lighting, alarms.
- Install an alarm system that fits your home and family needs.

Helpful ideas:

Do not use oxygen absorbers when storing sugar. It becomes a brick. It is still usable, just more difficult.

Oxygen absorbers may also cause your grains to not sprout (sprouting is a great way to get fresh green and enzymes from your storage).

Unflavored shortening unopened, has an almost indefinite storage life. Olive oil has a very long shelf-life when kept in a cool temperature and out of light.

Your mylar emergency blanket may be used in a lot of different ways. Be creative.

Old prescriptions get weaker and dosage cannot be guaranteed, but may be better than nothing in a TRUE EMERGENCY ONLY! The exceptions to this are Tetracycline and Doxycycline which become TOXIC.

Learn to use and rely on your herbal remedies.

Things to do with a safety pin:

1. Replace broken zipper or button on tents, clothing and sleeping bags.
2. Pin gloves to jacket arms.
3. Pop blisters.
4. Fishhook
5. Unclog stove
6. Neurosensory scan
7. Remove splinters
8. Replace lost screws in glasses
9. Clean rusty battery cables
10. Fix ski binding
11. Pin jacket or shirt arm to fashion a shoulder immobilizer
12. Poke holes in cardboard to fashion glasses or watch a solar eclipse
13. Leather punch
14. Emergency sewing device
15. Dressing fastener when out of tape
16. Punch holes in plastic bag for shower or irrigating bag

THINKING AHEAD

1. Educate yourself and your family.
   - Learn what disasters and hazards are common in your area.
   - Learn where evacuation shelters are located and local evacuation routes.
   - Learn your disaster plan at work and schools, including how to reunite with your children

2. Create a family emergency plan.
   - Have a family meeting to create an emergency plan and make sure everyone knows the plan.
   - Develop two routes to get out of your house.
   - Develop and identify safe places in your home.
   - Identify a place for your family to meet in case you are separated.
   - Identify a contact person outside of your immediate area.
   - Provide for safety for your pets.
   - Develop and update your 72-hour emergency and emotional emergency kits.
   - Know how to turn off electricity and gas and water to your home.

3. Have a family communication plan.
   - Make sure family members know emergency phone numbers and contacts.
   - Practice escape routes for multiple emergencies.

4. Make an emergency supply kit.
   - Think ahead. Do not build a kit that cannot be moved easily. Store your supply in a secure, yet accessible place.
   - Food and water. One gallon of water per day per person. Meals that take a minimum amount of preparation. Utensils for cooking and eating and shelter. Food and water for pets.
   - One warm blanket (mylar) for each person.
   - Tools. Flashlights/batteries. Portable radio/batteries. Wrench, small hammer, hatchet, knife, string or fishing line, safety pins.
   - First-aid kit. Add prescription medications. Emotional first-aid kit: items that appeal to the senses to provide comfort from anxiety – something to look at,

something to smell, something to touch, something to listen to, something to taste. Include cards, a book, coloring supplies.

- Sanitation supplies. Toilet paper, tissues, feminine products, wipes, soap or gel, trash bags.
- Extras. Car and house keys, important documents, cash and/or debit-credit cards.

5. Be informed.
- Keep informed about risk and safety information on radio, TV, and internet, including any hotline phone numbers.

6. Practice.
- Every six months:
Update and refresh your emergency supply kit. Put it on your calendar so you don't forget.
Review your disaster plan with the whole family.
- Once a year:
Practice your family emergency plan(s)
Update and refresh your emergency supply kit. Put it on your calendar so you don't forget.

Tips for using a Portable Generator

1. Always read and follow manufacturer's operating instructions.
2. Engines emit carbon monoxide. Never use a generator inside your home, garage, crawl space, or other enclosed areas. When fatal fumes build up, fans and open doors or windows do not provide enough fresh air.
3. Only use your generator outdoors.
4. Gasoline and its vapors are extremely flammable. Allow the generator engine to cool at least 2 minutes before refueling. Always use fresh gasoline.
5. If you use extension cords, uncoil them because of heat and only use grounded cords.
6. If you are connecting your generator to your home, have an electrician install a Power Transfer Switch. Never plug the generator directly into your home outlet.
7. Protect your generator from the weather.

Generator Sizes

1. Small portable: 2,000 to 4,000 watts; about $500 to $1,000.
   Powers the basics, such as: refrigerator, microwave, sump pump, several lights, TV.

2. Midsized portable/Small stationary: 5,000 to 8,500 watts; $800 to 1,500.
   Powers same as small models plus:
   Portable heater (1,300 watts), computer, heating system (500 watts), second pump, more lights.

3. Large portable: 10,000 watts; about $3,000 to $5,000.
   Powers same as midsized plus:
   Small water heater (3,000 watts), Central air conditioner (5,000 watts), electric stove.

4. Large Stationary: 10,000 to 15,000 watts; $4,000 to $10,000 or more, plus installation.
   Powers same as large portable model plus:
   Clothes washer and electric dryer.

PSYCHOLOGICAL SAFETY

Connecting With Other People
1. Social Support
   Seek someone to help or talk to
   Find a time and place where you won't be interrupted
   Brainstorm positive ways to cope
   Plan another time to talk

2. Psychological First Aid
   Professional support after a disaster or crisis
   Reduction of initial distress
   Support of short- and long-term functioning to adapt to trauma

3. When Awful Things Happen
   Immediate Reactions

Domain	Negative Responses	Positive Responses
Cognitive	Confusion, Disorientation, Worry, Intrusive Thoughts and Images, Guilt and Self-Blame	Determined, Resolved, Sharp Perspective of Details, Courage, Optimism, Faith
Emotional	Shock, Sorrow, Grief, Worry, Fear, Anger, Numbness, Irritability, Shame	Getting Involved, Challenging, Motivated
Social	Extreme Withdrawal, interpersonal Conflict	Social Connections, Alturistic, Helping Others
Physiological	Fatigue, Headache, Muscle Tension, Stomachache, Elevated Heart Rate, Disturbed Sleep, Exaggerated Startle Response	Alert, Ready to Respond, Energetic

What things don't help:

    Using alcohol or drugs to cope

    Working more

    Avoiding thinking or talking about your trauma

    Violence

    Overeating or not eating at all

    Highly risky behaviors

    Blaming other people

4. Emotional First Aid

    Build a Kit to Soothe the Senses

    Touch: Soft Material, Rock, Piece of Smooth Wood, Coin, etc.

    Smell: Potpourri, candle, Perfume, etc.

    Taste: Mint, Gum, Candy, Chocolate, etc.

    Hearing: CD, Tibetan Bowl, Tuning fork, etc.

    Sight: Picture, Image, etc.

5. After the Trauma/Crisis

    Stay around people who are positive and care about you.

    Tell someone about the problems you are facing.

    Stay active and Keep Busy.

    CDC.Gov

PART SEVEN

FOODS, BOTH WILD AND DOMESTICATED OR GROWN BY YOUR OWN HAND

FOODS

HERB	PART	PREPARATION
Cattails	Root	Grind/Powder into flour
	Bulb	Use as potato, cooked, use as cucumber raw
	New stalks	Use as rhubarb
	Heads	Use as insulation or chinking
Wild Barley, Oats	Seed	Grind/Powder into flour
Grass	Seed	Grind/Powder into flour
	Blade	Chew for moisture
Bulrushes	Root	Grind/Powder into flour
Wild Onions	Bulb	Eat raw or use for cooking
	Stem	
Mustard	Leaves	Boil as greens
	Seeds	Grind/Powder and make into paste for condiment
Nasturtiums	Flower	Eat raw in salad
	Leaves	
Marigolds	Flower	Soup spice
Dandelions	Young Flowers	Use as mushrooms
	Young leaves	Use as greens, cooked or raw in salad
Mushrooms	Fungus	Cook as desired, after testing for toxicity
Comfrey	Leaves	Salad
Alfalfa	Seeds	Grind/Powder into flour
	Sprouts	Salad additive
Anise	Leaves	Salad additive
	Stalks	
Plantain	Seeds	Grind/Powder into flour
Sassafras	Roots	Mild drink (similar to root beer)
Summer Savory	Whole Plant	Spice
Wild Strawberry, Blueberry, or Raspberry	Berry	Fruit

Nettles	New leaves	Boil as greens
Burdock	New leaves	Boil as greens
	New stalks	Eat as rhubarb
Queen Anne's Lace	Root	Eat as carrots, cooked or raw
Maple Syrup	Maple Sap	Eat as syrup

MEATS AND HIDE PREPARATIONS

JERKED MEATS:

5# of meat, sliced 1/8 inch thick, 3-4 inches wide.

¾ cup pineapple juice

¾ cup soya sauce

¼ cup brown sugar

2 Tablespoons molasses

3 Tablespoons Worcestershire sauce

1 Tablespoon Kosher salt

1 Tablespoon Thyme

1 ½ teaspoon Red Pepper

¾ teaspoon Allspice

Optional Spices: ¾ cup Teriyaki sauce

1 ½ teaspoon Cayenne Pepper

¾ teaspoon Nutmeg

Oven/Smoker:

1. Mix spices well and put into a container that will hold the meat.
2. Add the meat and make sure it is all well-covered with the sauce. Refrigerate for 8-12 hours.
3. Preheat oven to 175° F.
   Pat meat dry and place on a wire rack or smoker rack.
   Throw away remaining marinade.
4. Bake/Smoke for 2 hours.
5. Flip meat strips and bake/smoke another 2-2 ½ hours or until the surface is dry.

Dehydrating:

1. Mix spices well and put into a container that will hold the meat.
2. Add the meat and make sure it is all covered with the sauce. Refrigerate for 8-12 hours.
3. Turn on dehydrator to 160° F. and place meat evenly on the racks.
4. Dehydrate for 2 hours.
5. Turn dehydrator to 155° F. and flip meat over.
6. Dehydrate for 3 hours or until meat surface is dry.

Store jerked meat in the refrigerator. Eat and enjoy at your leisure.

CANNED MEATS

Poultry:

Clean well and cut into halves or quarters.

Foil poultry meat until about ½ done.

Stuff hot, into quart or ½ gallon jars and add 1 teaspoon salt for quarts, 1 ½ teaspoons salt for ½ gallons

Fill jar to within 1-inch of rim with hot broth.

Remove air bubbles.

Adjust cap and lid.

Process quarts for 1 hour and 30 minutes at 10 pounds pressure in a pressure canner.

Process ½ gallons for 2 hours at 10 pounds pressure in a pressure canner.

Beef, Pork, Venison, Bear, Buffalo or Elk:

Use quart-sized jars.

Cut meat into jar-sized chunks. Roast meat until it is well-browned.

Stuff jars with hot meat and add 1 teaspoon salt.

Cover with hot gravy or broth, leaving 1-inch head space.

Remove air bubbles.

Adjust cap and lid.

Process quarts for 1 hour and 30 minutes at 10 pounds pressure in a pressure canner.

Wild rabbit or squirrel (woodchuck, beaver tail, etc.):

Soak the meat for 1 hour in brine made by dissolving 1 Tablespoon salt per quart of water. Rinse.

Cut meat into quarters and de-bone. Boil meat until it is about ½ done.

Stuff hot, into quart jars.

Fill jar to within 1 inch of rim with hot broth.

Omit salt.

Process quarts for 1 hours and 30 minutes at 10 pounds pressure in a pressure canner.

Gravy to use in hot packing:

Remove meat from cook pot. Add 1 cup boiling water or broth for each 1 to 2 Tablespoons fat in pan.

Boil for 2-3 minutes. DO NOT THICKEN.

Salmon, Haddock or Trout:

Dissolve 2 cup salt in 1 gallon of water to make brine.

Cut fish into jar-length strips.

Cover fish well in the brine and let stand 2 hours.

Drain for 20 minutes.

Pack fish into jars, skin side next to the glass.

Leave a 1-inch head space.

Adjust lid and ring.

Process 1 hour and 40 minutes at 10 pounds pressure in a pressure canner.

CURING BACON AT HOME:

Mix together: 5# of PORK belly meat.
                   ¼ cup sea salt or pink salt
                   ½ cup pure cane sugar
                   1 Tablespoon black pepper

Coat meat evenly. Refrigerate 5 days, turning over daily.

Wash, dry and wrap in cheesecloth. Refrigerate 2 more days.

Rub meat with hickory salt or desired spices.

Smoke at 175° - 200° F. for 3 hours (internal temperature should be at least 150° F.)

Wrap and refrigerate for 8 hours.

Slice, package and freeze or cook.

CURING HAM AT HOME:
WET CURE:
Brine: 4 gallons of water (or enough to completely cover the ham portion in a five-gallon pail).
1 ½ cups Kosher Salt
1 ½ cups brown sugar
3 Tablespoons Prague Powder
1 Tablespoon pink salt
Mix well until all ingredients are dissolved.

Submerge meat in the brine. Keep the brining meat cold.
Turn over every day for the first week.
Cure for a total of 1 month, turning every 4 days until finished.
Bake and eat or smoke for added flavor.

To smoke: Rinse off and pat dry.
Rub with hickory salt or other desired spices.
Smoke for 5 hours or until internal temperature is 170° F.
Cut and eat, bake to desired taste, or freeze.

SMOKE CURE:
2 full pork "hams"
Rinse and pat dry.
Rub well with hickory smoke spice or other desired spices.
Fill water pan with ½ apple juice and ½ water and put in bottom of smoker.
Place desired smoker wood into a pan and place on smoker rack.
When wood begins to smoke, it is time to put the meat into the smoker.
Put in smoker for 4 hours or until internal temperature is 170° F.
Turn meat over hourly. Refill the water pan and wood chips as needed.

SURVIVAL

89

If using the oven, fill a pan with ½ cup apple juice and ½ cup water and place in the bottom of the oven.

Place desired smoker wood into a pan and place on the bottom rack of the oven.

Place the rubbed meat on a foil-lined pan on the top rack of the oven.

When the wood begins to smoke, it is time to put the meat into the oven.

Bake at 300° F. for 4 hours or until internal temperature is at least 160° F.

Turn meat over hourly.

Do not allow wood or water to dissipate. Refill as needed.

Remove meat and rub surface with butter to form a sheen. Bake at 350° F. until internal temperature is 170° F. (about ½ to ¾ hour).

Wrap and freeze or cut and eat.

BUTCHERING GUIDES

Beef Chart

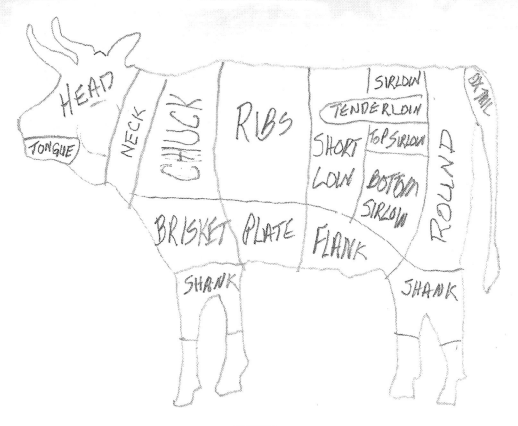

BEEF

Pork and Bear Charts

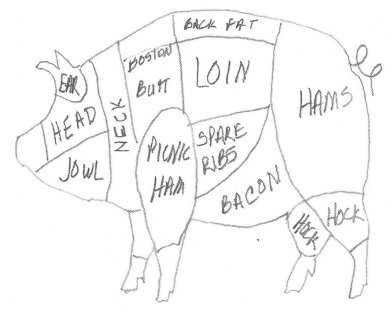

PORK

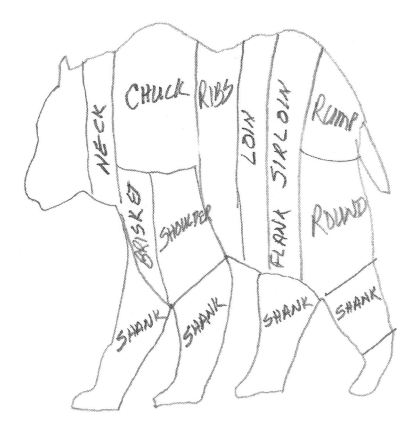

BEAR

Lamb and Deer Charts

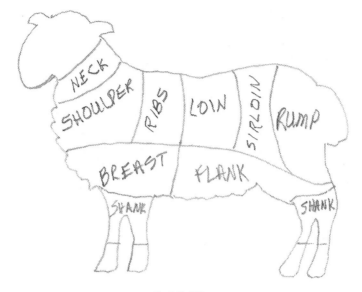

LAMB

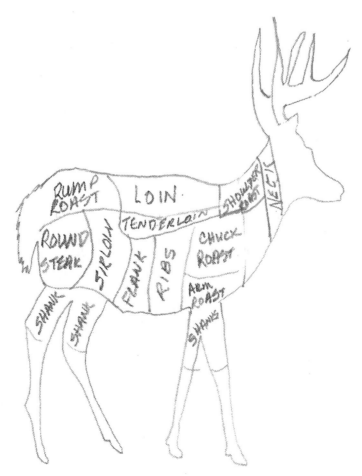

MOOSE, DEER, ELK

Rabbit, Squirrel and other Rodents Charts

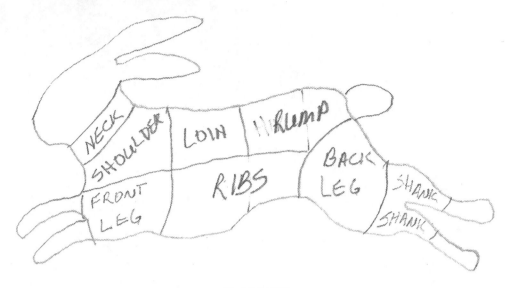

RABBIT

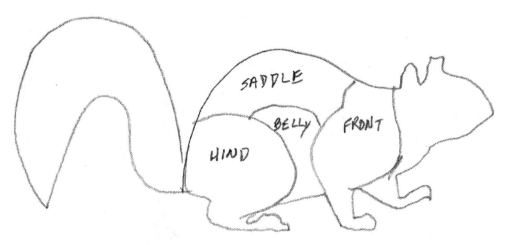

SQUIRREL and other Rodents

Poultry Charts
(Chicken, Duck, Goose, Turkey)

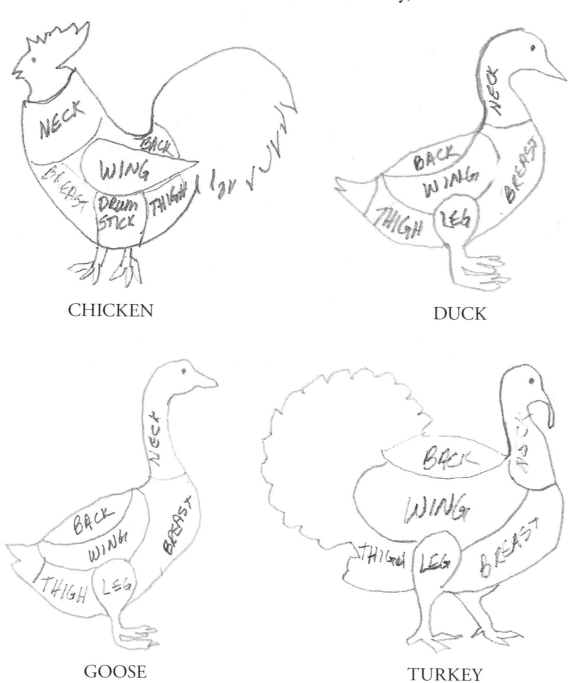

CHICKEN

DUCK

GOOSE

TURKEY

Fish, Frog and Turtle Charts

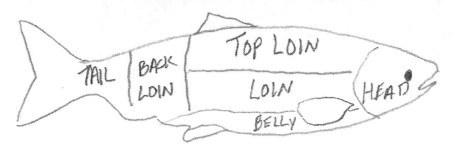

FISH

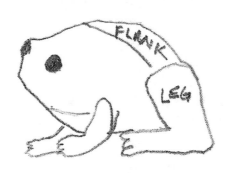

FROG

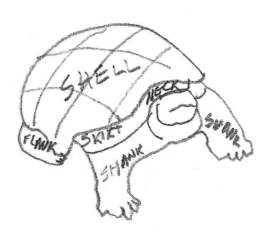

TURTLE

TANNING HIDES WITH ANIMAL BRAINS

Step One / Skinning and Fleshing:

After the animal is skinned, the hide **MUST BE CAREFULLY FLESHED** to remove any leftover fat and tissue.

This is done by scraping the inside of the hide to remove ALL flesh, fat, and tissue residue.

Step Two / Initial Soaking:

The hide must be **soaked in water** for three days. This allows the hair to slip or loosen, and raises and softens the grain layer of the hide. If it is not soaked sufficiently, the grain will not raise and the hide will not soften properly. However, if you are leaving the hair on the hide, this step will be skipped.

Step Three / Graining:

After the hair begins to slip, the hide must be **thoroughly scraped to remove all the hair, the follicles, and a portion of the grain, or the outer layer of the hide.** (*Skip this step if you are leaving the hair on*). This can be the most intensive step of the process – labor intensive.

Step Four / Membraning:

This critical step involves **removing the first layer of mucous membrane from the fleshy side of the skin.** (*Skip if you are leaving on the hair*). If the membrane is not removed, the brain mixture won't be able to penetrate the skin and your hide will not get soft.

Insure that you have **COMPLETELY** cleaned the <u>inner side</u> of the hide if you are leaving the hair on the outside. The outside must also be dirt- and bug-free, especially at the skin level.

Step Five / Wringing

Wringing helps further to break down the mucous membrane and, done properly, leaves the hide with the appropriate water content for maximum flexibility. This is usually accomplished by **attaching the hide to an anchor point (like nailing it to a post) and then twisting it around a large stick to remove as much water as possible**. Anchor the twisted hide to the post. This process takes 4-6 weeks. You must wring it again two to three times per week to maximize the twist and flexibility. Alternate the twist, first one way and the next time the other way.

TANNING HIDES WITH ANIMAL BRAINS, CONTINUED

Step Six / Braining

Animal brains are heated in water (1 pound of brain per gallon of water). It takes one pound of brain for a medium hide. The braining solution must have the consistency of "a brain milkshake".

A note to the squeamish: eggs, oil, and soap in equal amounts will also work, although not as well as brains. Also, you must rub the brains into the water *until it becomes the correct consistency.*

The water should be very warm, but not so hot that you can't put your hands into the brain solution. Put the skin in a tub containing the solution and **massage the hide by hand** to help the emulsifiers in the brain tissue penetrate the hide. This part takes a long time to do properly (2-3 hours is not unusual). Most hides take two brainings, but some may take up to five. Take your time with this step. Every inch of the hide must be rubbed with the brain (or egg) solution so that it penetrates evenly. Brain it once, then wring it for a day, changing the twist every three hours, then brain and wring it again (and again if need be) until it begins to feel soft and supple.

Step Seven / Hand Softening

This is critical to producing the soft, supple feel of traditional buckskin. After the final braining, the hide should be worked across a firm object (the backs of chairs or a board fence work well; you may also use a steel T-post). Properly softened, the hide should be supple even after it gets wet. After washing, the hide may take a bit of manual manipulation to soften completely, but it should take only a few minutes to make the clothing supple after a wash. This step was also done by chewing the hide to soften the material by native peoples and pioneers or "mountain men."

Step Eight / Smoking

Stitch two hides together and suspend them over a smoky fire or commercial smoker. The key is to use punky wood, which creates smoke without flame. The tent design traps the smoke in the hides and gives the finished buckskin a distinctive color and smell based on the wood used.

Sage leaves give the hide a yellow hue.

Douglas fir gives the skin a brown finish.

The smoke acts as a preservative.

Personal Notes:

REFERENCES

American Red Cross. Org, 2020

The Centers for Disease Control and Prevention, Atlanta, GA, 2004

The National Oceanic and Atmospheric Administration, Washington, DC

Standing Rules of Engagement, U.S. Military Home Defense Tactics, 1990.

Federal Emergency Management Agency, U. S. Department of Homeland Security, Washington, DC, 2012

National Safety Council, Itasca, IL, 2010

DEEP, Center for Disaster & Extreme Event Preparedness, 2004

CDC, U. S. Center for Disease Control and Prevention, *After the Storm,* 2004

Meat charts contain their references from stock photos.

Recipes and uses for herbs have been adapted by the author from native and indigenous peoples in the United States, Canada, and Mexico. All formulas have been used and/or modified by the author with success. Any similarities to other formulas or recipes is purely coincidental.

THE END

Printed in the United States
by Baker & Taylor Publisher Services